50% OFF
Online CPHQ Prep Course!

By Mometrix University

Dear Customer,

We consider it an honor and a privilege that you chose our CPHQ Study Guide. As a way of showing our appreciation and to help us better serve you, we are offering **50% off our online CPHQ Prep Course.** Many CPHQ courses cost hundreds of dollars. As a valued customer, **you will only pay $19.99 each month**, which is 50% off our regular monthly price of $39.99.

We have structured our online course to perfectly complement your printed study guide. The CPHQ Prep Course contains **in-depth lessons** that cover all the most important topics, **video reviews** that explain difficult concepts, over **700 practice questions** to ensure you feel prepared, and more than **350 digital flashcards**, so you can study while you're on the go.

Online CPHQ Prep Course

Topics Covered:

- Organizational Leadership
  - Structure and Integration
  - Regulatory, Accreditation, and External Recognition
- Health Data Analytics
  - Design and Data Management
  - Measurement and Analysis
- Performance and Process Improvement
  - Identifying Opportunities for Improvement
  - Implementation and Evaluation
- Patient Safety
  - Assessment and Planning
  - Implementation and Evaluation

Course Features:

- CPHQ Study Guide
  - Get content that complements our best-selling study guide.
- Full-Length Practice Tests
  - With over 700 practice questions, you can test yourself again and again.
- Mobile Friendly
  - If you need to study on the go, the course is easily accessible from your mobile device.
- CPHQ Flashcards
  - Our course includes a flashcard mode consisting of over 350 content cards to help you study.

To receive this discount, visit our website: https://www.mometrix.com/university/courses/cphq and add the course to your cart. At the checkout page, enter the discount code: **cphq50off**

If you have any questions or concerns, please don't hesitate to contact us at universityhelp@mometrix.com.

Sincerely,

FREE Study Skills DVD Offer

Dear Customer,

Thank you for your purchase from Mometrix! We consider it an honor and a privilege that you have purchased our product and we want to ensure your satisfaction.

As a way of showing our appreciation and to help us better serve you, we have developed a Study Skills DVD that we would like to give you for <u>FREE</u>. This DVD covers our *best practices* for getting ready for your exam, from how to use our study materials to how to best prepare for the day of the test.

All that we ask is that you email us with feedback that would describe your experience so far with our product. Good, bad, or indifferent, we want to know what you think!

To get your FREE Study Skills DVD, email <u>freedvd@mometrix.com</u> with *FREE STUDY SKILLS DVD* in the subject line and the following information in the body of the email:

- The name of the product you purchased.
- Your product rating on a scale of 1-5, with 5 being the highest rating.
- Your feedback. It can be long, short, or anything in between. We just want to know your impressions and experience so far with our product. (Good feedback might include how our study material met your needs and ways we might be able to make it even better. You could highlight features that you found helpful or features that you think we should add.)
- Your full name and shipping address where you would like us to send your free DVD.

If you have any questions or concerns, please don't hesitate to contact me directly.

Thanks again!

Sincerely,

Jay Willis
Vice President
<u>jay.willis@mometrix.com</u>
1-800-673-8175

CPHQ

Study Guide
2020 and 2021

CHPQ Exam Secrets
Study Guide

Full-Length Practice Exam

Detailed Answer
Explanations

Written and edited by Mometrix Test Prep

Printed in the United States of America

This paper meets the requirements of ANSI/NISO Z39.48-1992 (Permanence of Paper).

Mometrix offers volume discount pricing to institutions. For more information or a price quote, please contact our sales department at sales@mometrix.com or 888-248-1219.

Mometrix Media LLC is not affiliated with or endorsed by any official testing organization. All organizational and test names are trademarks of their respective owners.

Paperback
ISBN 13: 978-1-5167-2085-9
ISBN 10: 1-5167-2085-7

DEAR FUTURE EXAM SUCCESS STORY

First of all, **THANK YOU** for purchasing Mometrix study materials!

Second, congratulations! You are one of the few determined test-takers who are committed to doing whatever it takes to excel on your exam. **You have come to the right place.** We developed these study materials with one goal in mind: to deliver you the information you need in a format that's concise and easy to use.

In addition to optimizing your guide for the content of the test, we've outlined our recommended steps for breaking down the preparation process into small, attainable goals so you can make sure you stay on track.

We've also analyzed the entire test-taking process, identifying the most common pitfalls and showing how you can overcome them and be ready for any curveball the test throws you.

Standardized testing is one of the biggest obstacles on your road to success, which only increases the importance of doing well in the high-pressure, high-stakes environment of test day. Your results on this test could have a significant impact on your future, and this guide provides the information and practical advice to help you achieve your full potential on test day.

Your success is our success

We would love to hear from you! If you would like to share the story of your exam success or if you have any questions or comments in regard to our products, please contact us at **800-673-8175** or **support@mometrix.com**.

Thanks again for your business and we wish you continued success!

Sincerely,
The Mometrix Test Preparation Team

Need more help? Check out our flashcards at:
http://MometrixFlashcards.com/CPHQ

TABLE OF CONTENTS

Introduction

Thank you for purchasing this resource! You have made the choice to prepare yourself for a test that could have a huge impact on your future, and this guide is designed to help you be fully ready for test day. Obviously, it's important to have a solid understanding of the test material, but you also need to be prepared for the unique environment and stressors of the test, so that you can perform to the best of your abilities.

For this purpose, the first section that appears in this guide is the **Secret Keys**. We've devoted countless hours to meticulously researching what works and what doesn't, and we've boiled down our findings to the five most impactful steps you can take to improve your performance on the test. We start at the beginning with study planning and move through the preparation process, all the way to the testing strategies that will help you get the most out of what you know when you're finally sitting in front of the test.

We recommend that you start preparing for your test as far in advance as possible. However, if you've bought this guide as a last-minute study resource and only have a few days before your test, we recommend that you skip over the first two Secret Keys since they address a long-term study plan.

If you struggle with **test anxiety**, we strongly encourage you to check out our recommendations for how you can overcome it. Test anxiety is a formidable foe, but it can be beaten, and we want to make sure you have the tools you need to defeat it.

1

Secret Key #1 – Plan Big, Study Small

There's a lot riding on your performance. If you want to ace this test, you're going to need to keep your skills sharp and the material fresh in your mind. You need a plan that lets you review everything you need to know while still fitting in your schedule. We'll break this strategy down into three categories.

Information Organization

Start with the information you already have: the official test outline. From this, you can make a complete list of all the concepts you need to cover before the test. Organize these concepts into groups that can be studied together, and create a list of any related vocabulary you need to learn so you can brush up on any difficult terms. You'll want to keep this vocabulary list handy once you actually start studying since you may need to add to it along the way.

Time Management

Once you have your set of study concepts, decide how to spread them out over the time you have left before the test. Break your study plan into small, clear goals so you have a manageable task for each day and know exactly what you're doing. Then just focus on one small step at a time. When you manage your time this way, you don't need to spend hours at a time studying. Studying a small block of content for a short period each day helps you retain information better and avoid stressing over how much you have left to do. You can relax knowing that you have a plan to cover everything in time. In order for this strategy to be effective though, you have to start studying early and stick to your schedule. Avoid the exhaustion and futility that comes from last-minute cramming!

Study Environment

The environment you study in has a big impact on your learning. Studying in a coffee shop, while probably more enjoyable, is not likely to be as fruitful as studying in a quiet room. It's important to keep distractions to a minimum. You're only planning to study for a short block of time, so make the most of it. Don't pause to check your phone or get up to find a snack. It's also important to **avoid multitasking**. Research has consistently shown that multitasking will make your studying dramatically less effective. Your study area should also be comfortable and well-lit so you don't have the distraction of straining your eyes or sitting on an uncomfortable chair.

The time of day you study is also important. You want to be rested and alert. Don't wait until just before bedtime. Study when you'll be most likely to comprehend and remember. Even better, if you know what time of day your test will be, set that time aside for study. That way your brain will be used to working on that subject at that specific time and you'll have a better chance of recalling information.

Finally, it can be helpful to team up with others who are studying for the same test. Your actual studying should be done in as isolated an environment as possible, but the work of organizing the information and setting up the study plan can be divided up. In between study sessions, you can discuss with your teammates the concepts that you're all studying and quiz each other on the details. Just be sure that your teammates are as serious about the test as you are. If you find that your study time is being replaced with social time, you might need to find a new team.

Secret Key #2 – Make Your Studying Count

You're devoting a lot of time and effort to preparing for this test, so you want to be absolutely certain it will pay off. This means doing more than just reading the content and hoping you can remember it on test day. It's important to make every minute of study count. There are two main areas you can focus on to make your studying count:

Retention

It doesn't matter how much time you study if you can't remember the material. You need to make sure you are retaining the concepts. To check your retention of the information you're learning, try recalling it at later times with minimal prompting. Try carrying around flashcards and glance at one or two from time to time or ask a friend who's also studying for the test to quiz you.

To enhance your retention, look for ways to put the information into practice so that you can apply it rather than simply recalling it. If you're using the information in practical ways, it will be much easier to remember. Similarly, it helps to solidify a concept in your mind if you're not only reading it to yourself but also explaining it to someone else. Ask a friend to let you teach them about a concept you're a little shaky on (or speak aloud to an imaginary audience if necessary). As you try to summarize, define, give examples, and answer your friend's questions, you'll understand the concepts better and they will stay with you longer. Finally, step back for a big picture view and ask yourself how each piece of information fits with the whole subject. When you link the different concepts together and see them working together as a whole, it's easier to remember the individual components.

Finally, practice showing your work on any multi-step problems, even if you're just studying. Writing out each step you take to solve a problem will help solidify the process in your mind, and you'll be more likely to remember it during the test.

Modality

Modality simply refers to the means or method by which you study. Choosing a study modality that fits your own individual learning style is crucial. No two people learn best in exactly the same way, so it's important to know your strengths and use them to your advantage.

For example, if you learn best by visualization, focus on visualizing a concept in your mind and draw an image or a diagram. Try color-coding your notes, illustrating them, or creating symbols that will trigger your mind to recall a learned concept. If you learn best by hearing or discussing information, find a study partner who learns the same way or read aloud to yourself. Think about how to put the information in your own words. Imagine that you are giving a lecture on the topic and record yourself so you can listen to it later.

For any learning style, flashcards can be helpful. Organize the information so you can take advantage of spare moments to review. Underline key words or phrases. Use different colors for different categories. Mnemonic devices (such as creating a short list in which every item starts with the same letter) can also help with retention. Find what works best for you and use it to store the information in your mind most effectively and easily.

Secret Key #3 – Practice the Right Way

Your success on test day depends not only on how many hours you put into preparing, but also on whether you prepared the right way. It's good to check along the way to see if your studying is paying off. One of the most effective ways to do this is by taking practice tests to evaluate your progress. Practice tests are useful because they show exactly where you need to improve. Every time you take a practice test, pay special attention to these three groups of questions:

- The questions you got wrong
- The questions you had to guess on, even if you guessed right
- The questions you found difficult or slow to work through

This will show you exactly what your weak areas are, and where you need to devote more study time. Ask yourself why each of these questions gave you trouble. Was it because you didn't understand the material? Was it because you didn't remember the vocabulary? Do you need more repetitions on this type of question to build speed and confidence? Dig into those questions and figure out how you can strengthen your weak areas as you go back to review the material.

Additionally, many practice tests have a section explaining the answer choices. It can be tempting to read the explanation and think that you now have a good understanding of the concept. However, an explanation likely only covers part of the question's broader context. Even if the explanation makes sense, **go back and investigate** every concept related to the question until you're positive you have a thorough understanding.

As you go along, keep in mind that the practice test is just that: practice. Memorizing these questions and answers will not be very helpful on the actual test because it is unlikely to have any of the same exact questions. If you only know the right answers to the sample questions, you won't be prepared for the real thing. **Study the concepts** until you understand them fully, and then you'll be able to answer any question that shows up on the test.

It's important to wait on the practice tests until you're ready. If you take a test on your first day of study, you may be overwhelmed by the amount of material covered and how much you need to learn. Work up to it gradually.

On test day, you'll need to be prepared for answering questions, managing your time, and using the test-taking strategies you've learned. It's a lot to balance, like a mental marathon that will have a big impact on your future. Like training for a marathon, you'll need to start slowly and work your way up. When test day arrives, you'll be ready.

Start with the strategies you've read in the first two Secret Keys—plan your course and study in the way that works best for you. If you have time, consider using multiple study resources to get different approaches to the same concepts. It can be helpful to see difficult concepts from more than one angle. Then find a good source for practice tests. Many times, the test website will suggest potential study resources or provide sample tests.

Practice Test Strategy

If you're able to find at least three practice tests, we recommend this strategy:

UNTIMED AND OPEN-BOOK PRACTICE

Take the first test with no time constraints and with your notes and study guide handy. Take your time and focus on applying the strategies you've learned.

TIMED AND OPEN-BOOK PRACTICE

Take the second practice test open-book as well, but set a timer and practice pacing yourself to finish in time.

TIMED AND CLOSED-BOOK PRACTICE

Take any other practice tests as if it were test day. Set a timer and put away your study materials. Sit at a table or desk in a quiet room, imagine yourself at the testing center, and answer questions as quickly and accurately as possible.

Keep repeating timed and closed-book tests on a regular basis until you run out of practice tests or it's time for the actual test. Your mind will be ready for the schedule and stress of test day, and you'll be able to focus on recalling the material you've learned.

Secret Key #4 – Pace Yourself

Once you're fully prepared for the material on the test, your biggest challenge on test day will be managing your time. Just knowing that the clock is ticking can make you panic even if you have plenty of time left. Work on pacing yourself so you can build confidence against the time constraints of the exam. Pacing is a difficult skill to master, especially in a high-pressure environment, so **practice is vital**.

Set time expectations for your pace based on how much time is available. For example, if a section has 60 questions and the time limit is 30 minutes, you know you have to average 30 seconds or less per question in order to answer them all. Although 30 seconds is the hard limit, set 25 seconds per question as your goal, so you reserve extra time to spend on harder questions. When you budget extra time for the harder questions, you no longer have any reason to stress when those questions take longer to answer.

Don't let this time expectation distract you from working through the test at a calm, steady pace, but keep it in mind so you don't spend too much time on any one question. Recognize that taking extra time on one question you don't understand may keep you from answering two that you do understand later in the test. If your time limit for a question is up and you're still not sure of the answer, mark it and move on, and come back to it later if the time and the test format allow. If the testing format doesn't allow you to return to earlier questions, just make an educated guess; then put it out of your mind and move on.

On the easier questions, be careful not to rush. It may seem wise to hurry through them so you have more time for the challenging ones, but it's not worth missing one if you know the concept and just didn't take the time to read the question fully. Work efficiently but make sure you understand the question and have looked at all of the answer choices, since more than one may seem right at first.

Even if you're paying attention to the time, you may find yourself a little behind at some point. You should speed up to get back on track, but do so wisely. Don't panic; just take a few seconds less on each question until you're caught up. Don't guess without thinking, but do look through the answer choices and eliminate any you know are wrong. If you can get down to two choices, it is often worthwhile to guess from those. Once you've chosen an answer, move on and don't dwell on any that you skipped or had to hurry through. If a question was taking too long, chances are it was one of the harder ones, so you weren't as likely to get it right anyway.

On the other hand, if you find yourself getting ahead of schedule, it may be beneficial to slow down a little. The more quickly you work, the more likely you are to make a careless mistake that will affect your score. You've budgeted time for each question, so don't be afraid to spend that time. Practice an efficient but careful pace to get the most out of the time you have.

Secret Key #5 – Have a Plan for Guessing

When you're taking the test, you may find yourself stuck on a question. Some of the answer choices seem better than others, but you don't see the one answer choice that is obviously correct. What do you do?

The scenario described above is very common, yet most test takers have not effectively prepared for it. Developing and practicing a plan for guessing may be one of the single most effective uses of your time as you get ready for the exam.

In developing your plan for guessing, there are three questions to address:

- When should you start the guessing process?
- How should you narrow down the choices?
- Which answer should you choose?

When to Start the Guessing Process

Unless your plan for guessing is to select C every time (which, despite its merits, is not what we recommend), you need to leave yourself enough time to apply your answer elimination strategies. Since you have a limited amount of time for each question, that means that if you're going to give yourself the best shot at guessing correctly, you have to decide quickly whether or not you will guess.

Of course, the best-case scenario is that you don't have to guess at all, so first, see if you can answer the question based on your knowledge of the subject and basic reasoning skills. Focus on the key words in the question and try to jog your memory of related topics. Give yourself a chance to bring the knowledge to mind, but once you realize that you don't have (or you can't access) the knowledge you need to answer the question, it's time to start the guessing process.

It's almost always better to start the guessing process too early than too late. It only takes a few seconds to remember something and answer the question from knowledge. Carefully eliminating wrong answer choices takes longer. Plus, going through the process of eliminating answer choices can actually help jog your memory.

Summary: Start the guessing process as soon as you decide that you can't answer the question based on your knowledge.

How to Narrow Down the Choices

The next chapter in this book (**Test-Taking Strategies**) includes a wide range of strategies for how to approach questions and how to look for answer choices to eliminate. You will definitely want to read those carefully, practice them, and figure out which ones work best for you. Here though, we're going to address a mindset rather than a particular strategy.

Your chances of guessing an answer correctly depend on how many options you are choosing from.

How many choices you have	How likely you are to guess correctly
5	20%
4	25%
3	33%
2	50%
1	100%

You can see from this chart just how valuable it is to be able to eliminate incorrect answers and make an educated guess, but there are two things that many test takers do that cause them to miss out on the benefits of guessing:

- Accidentally eliminating the correct answer
- Selecting an answer based on an impression

We'll look at the first one here, and the second one in the next section.

To avoid accidentally eliminating the correct answer, we recommend a thought exercise called **the $5 challenge**. In this challenge, you only eliminate an answer choice from contention if you are willing to bet $5 on it being wrong. Why $5? Five dollars is a small but not insignificant amount of money. It's an amount you could afford to lose but wouldn't want to throw away. And while losing $5 once might not hurt too much, doing it twenty times will set you back $100. In the same way, each small decision you make—eliminating a choice here, guessing on a question there—won't by itself impact your score very much, but when you put them all together, they can make a big difference. By holding each answer choice elimination decision to a higher standard, you can reduce the risk of accidentally eliminating the correct answer.

The $5 challenge can also be applied in a positive sense: If you are willing to bet $5 that an answer choice *is* correct, go ahead and mark it as correct.

Summary: Only eliminate an answer choice if you are willing to bet $5 that it is wrong.

Which Answer to Choose

You're taking the test. You've run into a hard question and decided you'll have to guess. You've eliminated all the answer choices you're willing to bet $5 on. Now you have to pick an answer. Why do we even need to talk about this? Why can't you just pick whichever one you feel like when the time comes?

The answer to these questions is that if you don't come into the test with a plan, you'll rely on your impression to select an answer choice, and if you do that, you risk falling into a trap. The test writers know that everyone who takes their test will be guessing on some of the questions, so they intentionally write wrong answer choices to seem plausible. You still have to pick an answer though, and if the wrong answer choices are designed to look right, how can you ever be sure that you're not falling for their trap? The best solution we've found to this dilemma is to take the decision out of your hands entirely. Here is the process we recommend:

Once you've eliminated any choices that you are confident (willing to bet $5) are wrong, select the first remaining choice as your answer.

Whether you choose to select the first remaining choice, the second, or the last, the important thing is that you use some preselected standard. Using this approach guarantees that you will not be enticed into selecting an answer choice that looks right, because you are not basing your decision on how the answer choices look.

This is not meant to make you question your knowledge. Instead, it is to help you recognize the difference between your knowledge and your impressions. There's a huge difference between thinking an answer is right because of what you know, and thinking an answer is right because it looks or sounds like it should be right.

Summary: To ensure that your selection is appropriately random, make a predetermined selection from among all answer choices you have not eliminated.

Test-Taking Strategies

This section contains a list of test-taking strategies that you may find helpful as you work through the test. By taking what you know and applying logical thought, you can maximize your chances of answering any question correctly!

It is very important to realize that every question is different and every person is different: no single strategy will work on every question, and no single strategy will work for every person. That's why we've included all of them here, so you can try them out and determine which ones work best for different types of questions and which ones work best for you.

Question Strategies

READ CAREFULLY

Read the question and answer choices carefully. Don't miss the question because you misread the terms. You have plenty of time to read each question thoroughly and make sure you understand what is being asked. Yet a happy medium must be attained, so don't waste too much time. You must read carefully, but efficiently.

CONTEXTUAL CLUES

Look for contextual clues. If the question includes a word you are not familiar with, look at the immediate context for some indication of what the word might mean. Contextual clues can often give you all the information you need to decipher the meaning of an unfamiliar word. Even if you can't determine the meaning, you may be able to narrow down the possibilities enough to make a solid guess at the answer to the question.

PREFIXES

If you're having trouble with a word in the question or answer choices, try dissecting it. Take advantage of every clue that the word might include. Prefixes and suffixes can be a huge help. Usually they allow you to determine a basic meaning. Pre- means before, post- means after, pro - is positive, de- is negative. From prefixes and suffixes, you can get an idea of the general meaning of the word and try to put it into context.

HEDGE WORDS

Watch out for critical hedge words, such as *likely, may, can, sometimes, often, almost, mostly, usually, generally, rarely,* and *sometimes.* Question writers insert these hedge phrases to cover every possibility. Often an answer choice will be wrong simply because it leaves no room for exception. Be on guard for answer choices that have definitive words such as *exactly* and *always.*

SWITCHBACK WORDS

Stay alert for *switchbacks.* These are the words and phrases frequently used to alert you to shifts in thought. The most common switchback words are *but, although,* and *however.* Others include *nevertheless, on the other hand, even though, while, in spite of, despite, regardless of.* Switchback words are important to catch because they can change the direction of the question or an answer choice.

FACE VALUE

When in doubt, use common sense. Accept the situation in the problem at face value. Don't read too much into it. These problems will not require you to make wild assumptions. If you have to go beyond creativity and warp time or space in order to have an answer choice fit the question, then you should move on and consider the other answer choices. These are normal problems rooted in reality. The applicable relationship or explanation may not be readily apparent, but it is there for you to figure out. Use your common sense to interpret anything that isn't clear.

Answer Choice Strategies

ANSWER SELECTION

The most thorough way to pick an answer choice is to identify and eliminate wrong answers until only one is left, then confirm it is the correct answer. Sometimes an answer choice may immediately seem right, but be careful. The test writers will usually put more than one reasonable answer choice on each question, so take a second to read all of them and make sure that the other choices are not equally obvious. As long as you have time left, it is better to read every answer choice than to pick the first one that looks right without checking the others.

ANSWER CHOICE FAMILIES

An answer choice family consists of two (in rare cases, three) answer choices that are very similar in construction and cannot all be true at the same time. If you see two answer choices that are direct opposites or parallels, one of them is usually the correct answer. For instance, if one answer choice says that quantity x increases and another either says that quantity x decreases (opposite) or says that quantity y increases (parallel), then those answer choices would fall into the same family. An answer choice that doesn't match the construction of the answer choice family is more likely to be incorrect. Most questions will not have answer choice families, but when they do appear, you should be prepared to recognize them.

ELIMINATE ANSWERS

Eliminate answer choices as soon as you realize they are wrong, but make sure you consider all possibilities. If you are eliminating answer choices and realize that the last one you are left with is also wrong, don't panic. Start over and consider each choice again. There may be something you missed the first time that you will realize on the second pass.

AVOID FACT TRAPS

Don't be distracted by an answer choice that is factually true but doesn't answer the question. You are looking for the choice that answers the question. Stay focused on what the question is asking for so you don't accidentally pick an answer that is true but incorrect. Always go back to the question and make sure the answer choice you've selected actually answers the question and is not merely a true statement.

EXTREME STATEMENTS

In general, you should avoid answers that put forth extreme actions as standard practice or proclaim controversial ideas as established fact. An answer choice that states the "process should be used in certain situations, if..." is much more likely to be correct than one that states the "process should be discontinued completely." The first is a calm rational statement and doesn't even make a definitive, uncompromising stance, using a hedge word *if* to provide wiggle room, whereas the second choice is a radical idea and far more extreme.

BENCHMARK

As you read through the answer choices and you come across one that seems to answer the question well, mentally select that answer choice. This is not your final answer, but it's the one that will help you evaluate the other answer choices. The one that you selected is your benchmark or standard for judging each of the other answer choices. Every other answer choice must be compared to your benchmark. That choice is correct until proven otherwise by another answer choice beating it. If you find a better answer, then that one becomes your new benchmark. Once you've decided that no other choice answers the question as well as your benchmark, you have your final answer.

PREDICT THE ANSWER

Before you even start looking at the answer choices, it is often best to try to predict the answer. When you come up with the answer on your own, it is easier to avoid distractions and traps because you will know exactly what to look for. The right answer choice is unlikely to be word-for-word what you came up with, but it should be a close match. Even if you are confident that you have the right answer, you should still take the time to read each option before moving on.

General Strategies

TOUGH QUESTIONS

If you are stumped on a problem or it appears too hard or too difficult, don't waste time. Move on! Remember though, if you can quickly check for obviously incorrect answer choices, your chances of guessing correctly are greatly improved. Before you completely give up, at least try to knock out a couple of possible answers. Eliminate what you can and then guess at the remaining answer choices before moving on.

CHECK YOUR WORK

Since you will probably not know every term listed and the answer to every question, it is important that you get credit for the ones that you do know. Don't miss any questions through careless mistakes. If at all possible, try to take a second to look back over your answer selection and make sure you've selected the correct answer choice and haven't made a costly careless mistake (such as marking an answer choice that you didn't mean to mark). This quick double check should more than pay for itself in caught mistakes for the time it costs.

PACE YOURSELF

It's easy to be overwhelmed when you're looking at a page full of questions; your mind is confused and full of random thoughts, and the clock is ticking down faster than you would like. Calm down and maintain the pace that you have set for yourself. Especially as you get down to the last few minutes of the test, don't let the small numbers on the clock make you panic. As long as you are on track by monitoring your pace, you are guaranteed to have time for each question.

DON'T RUSH

It is very easy to make errors when you are in a hurry. Maintaining a fast pace in answering questions is pointless if it makes you miss questions that you would have gotten right otherwise. Test writers like to include distracting information and wrong answers that seem right. Taking a little extra time to avoid careless mistakes can make all the difference in your test score. Find a pace that allows you to be confident in the answers that you select.

KEEP MOVING

Panicking will not help you pass the test, so do your best to stay calm and keep moving. Taking deep breaths and going through the answer elimination steps you practiced can help to break through a stress barrier and keep your pace.

Final Notes

The combination of a solid foundation of content knowledge and the confidence that comes from practicing your plan for applying that knowledge is the key to maximizing your performance on test day. As your foundation of content knowledge is built up and strengthened, you'll find that the strategies included in this chapter become more and more effective in helping you quickly sift through the distractions and traps of the test to isolate the correct answer.

Now it's time to move on to the test content chapters of this book, but be sure to keep your goal in mind. As you read, think about how you will be able to apply this information on the test. If you've already seen sample questions for the test and you have an idea of the question format and style, try to come up with questions of your own that you can answer based on what you're reading. This will give you valuable practice applying your knowledge in the same ways you can expect to on test day.

Good luck and good studying!

14

Why Certify?

CPHQ

CPHQ stands for Certified Professional in Healthcare Quality. Certification is profitable to:

- Raise the standards in your field and distinguish your experience.
- Use your credentials to further your career.
- Improve your skills and abilities to manage workers

Score

In addition to the 125 scored questions, CPHQ examinations also include an additional 15 pretest questions. You will not be able to distinguish the scored questions from the pretest questions, and your performance on the pretest questions will not contribute to your score.

The CPHQ uses the following percentage guidelines in selecting the three types of questions that appear on each examination: 32% recall, 53% application, and 15% analysis. Recall questions test the candidate's knowledge of specific facts and concepts. Application questions require the candidate to interpret or apply information to a situation. Analysis questions test the candidate's ability to evaluate, problem solve or integrate a variety of information and/or judgment into a meaningful whole.

Scores are reported in written form only, in person or by U.S. mail. The score report will reflect either "pass" or "fail," followed by a raw score indicating the number of questions you answered correctly. Additional detail is provided in the form of raw scores by each of the four major content categories. This information is provided as feedback to help you understand your performance within the major content categories. Your pass/fail status is determined by your overall raw score for the entire examination.

Seven Pillars of Quality

SEVEN PILLARS OF QUALITY	
1. Efficacy 2. Effectiveness 3. Efficiency 4. Acceptability	Humanistic Outcomes
5. Optimality 6. Equity 7. Legitimacy	Society Outcomes

1. EFFICACY

This deals with a **controlled environment** and examines what is possible. It sets an upper boundary for quality and establishes the ideal to which all should aspire. However, as we know, the real world is very different to the laboratory. It is likely that the less control that is exerted over the environment, the less probable it is that practitioners are able to meet these standards.

2. EFFECTIVENESS

The second pillar of quality is *effectiveness* i.e. to what extent does the service achieve its **intended outcomes** in a real-world environment? Social, economic and individual factors influence the selection of quality indicators. Various indicators have been developed such as cost effective, socially effective and individually effective although the way in which they are measured is not always universally agreed.

3. EFFICIENCY

The third pillar of quality is *efficiency*. This examines the extent to which scarce resources are used to derive the **greatest benefits** with the **least waste**. This is usually measured by examining the ratio between the costs and benefits of a service and comparing these with others who are providing the same or similar services. This measure is typically used by socioeconomic forces seeking to select a service which will result in reduced costs. The assumption is made that the benefit stays the same, an assumption that is frequently not tested.

4. ACCEPTABILITY

The fourth pillar is *acceptability*. This concentrates on the usefulness of the service to the patient and its perceived impact on his/ her **quality of life**. It takes into consideration patient preferences regarding access to the service (e.g. advice), relationship with health service providers (egg trust, confidentiality), the amenities in which the service is provided and the cost utility relationship.

5. OPTIMALITY

The fifth pillar is *optimality*. From the point of view of society and the economic system, it is necessary to ensure that the **optimum allocation of resources** is achieved relative to the benefits derived from the services provided. Techniques such as cost benefit analysis and marginal costing are used to identify the optimum point of resource allocation: benefits. Quality indicators are usually of a global socioeconomic nature. Neither the individual service provider nor patient are concerned with these indicators. However, data collection starts at the interface between the two and the desire for maximal rather than optimal benefits may adversely influence the selection of appropriate indicators.

16

6. Equity

The sixth pillar is *equity*. Society is concerned that every person should receive **equal treatment**, or at best fair treatment. Equity is compromised when the quality of service or even the range of services is determined by the patient's ability to pay for the service. Since third party payers play a significant role in the health care system, equity would be affected by the extent to which a third-party payer includes a fee for the service in the benefits that it offers it members.

7. Legitimacy

The seventh and final pillar is *legitimacy*. This is similar to the concept of acceptability except that "the preferences and values for legitimacy are expressed through a **societal** rather than an individual perspective". Clearly, society requires evidence upon which to make these judgments.

Organizational Leadership

Structure and Integration

CERTIFIED PROFESSIONAL IN HEALTHCARE QUALITY

The **Certified Professional in Healthcare Quality** (CPHQ) has a unique and broad responsibility in an organization. The CPHQ promotes and supports quality assurance, safety, and effective healthcare. The quality professional must have the expertise to design, implement, and evaluate **process improvement activities**. The CPHQ must:

- Develop data collection and measurement procedures in order to evaluate outcomes.
- Provide education for administration and staff.
- Coordinate activities related to licensure, accreditation, standards, and regulations.
- Provide leadership as an agent of change within the organization.
- Identify organizational needs and opportunities for improvement.
- Prepare organization-wide plans, including quality management, patient safety, utilization and risk management.
- Document activities and provide summary reports to leadership and the governing board.
- Facilitate interdisciplinary participation and teams.
- Differentiate a variety of organizational needs.

TIME MANAGEMENT TECHNIQUES

Time management is an important function of leaders who must not only manage their own time, but must also model time management and schedule others' time effectively. Steps for effective time management are:

1. *Plan*: Create goals. Establish schedules for yearly, monthly, and daily activities. Plan each day in advance.
2. *Create a task list*: Update this task list daily, including routine tasks, so that all can be completed.
3. *Prioritize*: Rank the order in which tasks are to be accomplished, beginning with high priority items.
4. *Minimize paper handling*: Handle a paper or task once, instead of shuffling it about and dealing with it repeatedly.
5. *Use time effectively*: Avoid wasted time by starting meetings on schedule and ask a timekeeper to monitor the time and announce when the time is up. Work efficiently, paying attention to necessary details.
6. *Delegate*: Determine which tasks can be delegated to others and do not micromanage them.
7. *Use computer technology*: Avoid paper when possible. Keep calendars and lists on the computer for easy updating. Use e-mail and the Internet.
8. Avoid procrastination: Just do it.

ORGANIZATION-WIDE STRATEGIC PLANNING

Organization-wide strategic planning requires that an organization examines its needs, community, and customers and establishes goals for the *near future* (2–4 years) and the *extended future* (10–15 years). Strategic planning must be based on assessments, both internal and external, to determine the present courses of action, needed changes, priorities, and methodologies to effect

18

change. The focus of strategic planning must be on development of services. The organization identifies customer needs, develops services, and then markets those services.

Organization-wide strategic planning includes:

- Collecting data and doing an external analysis of customer needs in relation to regulations and demographics.
- Analyzing internal services and functions.
- Identifying and understanding key issues, including the strengths and weaknesses of the organization, potential opportunities, and negative impacts.
- Developing revised mission and vision statements that identify core values.
- Establishing specific goals and objectives, based on findings.

STRATEGIC QUALITY PLANNING TO PROMOTE PERFORMANCE IMPROVEMENT

Strategic quality planning to promote performance improvement must begin at the top level of management, with a commitment to facilitate change at all levels, and to provide the financial resources that make these changes possible. Every strategic quality plan begins with a clear *definition of quality* as it applies to customers, and relates this to the organization's mission and vision statements, goals, and objectives. Processes are redesigned to achieve quality. Organizational performance measurements are modified to ensure regulatory compliance. *Total quality management* (TQM) is at the center of all planning. An organization-wide model for quality performance must be used that includes at least the following:

- Assessment
- Planning
- Implementation
- Evaluation of continuous improvement

The planning process must be documented and must contain an *action plan* that ensures ongoing evaluation of progress.

CUSTOMER NEEDS AND SATISFACTION

Customer needs and satisfaction can be difficult to define because they are very individualized. Build an assessment of satisfaction, including opportunities for feedback, into any strategic plan. Patients are considered *external customers*. Patients want to avoid complications and regain their health without worrying about a plan. The *internal customers* include:

- *Hospital administrators,* who want a cost-effective plan, increased productivity, and reduced liability.
- *Physicians*, who want to provide positive outcomes for patients, and assistance in providing care.
- *Nurses* who want a practical, efficient plan that can be implemented without increasing their workload.
- *Environmental Services workers* want a plan that relates to the resources available in each department.
- *Accreditation agencies* want a plan providing documented proof of the organization's compliance with accreditation standards.
- *Communities/community agencies* want a plan that meets the needs of the various populations they represent.

- **Insurance companies** want a cost-saving plan.
- **Suppliers** want a profitable, efficient plan.

ORGANIZATIONAL ETHICS

Organizational ethics is the value system at work within an organization. While almost all healthcare organizations have a written Code of Ethics, an ethical organization embodies that code within all processes, including:

- A code of right conduct governing staff relationships with patients and the public.
- Recognition of the patient's right to quality care and respect for personal religious beliefs, culture, and psychosocial values.
- Transparency in disclosure of information, and accountability.
- Adherence to regulations and best practices.
- Recognition of the need to empower staff and patients.
- Leadership without intimidation or fear tactics.
- Standard, open guidelines for organ donation, procurement, and research projects.
- Maintenance of a bioethics committee to provide guidance related to ethical issues in healthcare.

> **Review Video: Organizational Ethics**
> Visit mometrix.com/academy and enter code: 885880

DEVELOPING AN ORGANIZATIONAL VISION STATEMENT

An **organizational vision statement** requires the CPHQ to analyze both **internal** and **external customer-supplier relationships**, so a statement about what the organization intends to become can be created. The vision statement is the commitment that the organization is making to its stakeholders. The vision statement outlines **future goals**, rather than focusing on what has already been achieved. Make the vision statement in one sentence or a short paragraph, for example:

Hospital X will be the leader in providing sustainable quality patient-centered care to (name the community), and to improve the physical and mental health of community members.

Follow the vision statement with an **explanation of terms**, so that such concepts as "sustainable" and "patient-centered" are clarified for the reader. For example, if "sustainable" is part of the vision statement, then the explanation should include "the need to function within budget constraints, while providing optimum care."

DEVELOPING AN ORGANIZATIONAL MISSION STATEMENT

The **mission statement** of an organization reflects the current status of the organization and describes, in broad terms, the **purpose** of the organization and its **role** in the community. Develop the mission statement in response to data and program analysis, and with input from all members of the organization. The mission statement identifies the organization or program, states its function, and outlines its purpose and strategy of the program, for example:

Hospital X is a collaborative group of professionals, physicians, administrators, nurses, and support staff. The mission of Hospital X is to promote the health and safety of its patients, visitors, and staff, and to provide outstanding quality health care services to (name the community).

The mission statement should in some way include a ***commitment to quality and patient care***, and the need to ***serve the community***. In many cases, the mission statement is followed by detailed explanations, which may include statements of organizational values, philosophy, and history.

DEVELOPING GOALS AND OBJECTIVES

Goals and objectives support the **mission and vision statements**, so complete them at the same time to determine if the mission and vision statements can be realized, and explain how that will happen.

Goals should be achievable aims, essentially end results, developed for specific units of the organization or the organization in general, focusing on improving performance. An example of a specific goal is:

- The Neonatal Intensive Care Unit will reduce surgical site infections by 30% from 2016 levels.
- In healthcare quality management, the goals must be based on knowledge about functions and processes within the organization, and **prioritized** accordingly, as part of achieving positive patient outcomes.

Objectives are the measurable steps taken to achieve goals, and in the case of infections, an objective might include:

- An Infection Control practitioner will audit antibiotic use, and the Physicians' Internal Medicine Committee will establish an antibiotic prophylaxis protocol within 6 months.
- Objectives must be measurable, include a **timeline**, and identify who is **responsible** for achieving the objective.

ENGAGING STAKEHOLDERS TO PROMOTE QUALITY AND SAFETY

PROMOTING QUALITY AND SAFETY THROUGH DISASTER/EMERGENCY PREPAREDNESS PLANS

Disaster/emergency preparedness plans should be in place based on the Hospital Emergency Incident Command System (HEICS), which provides a model for management, responsibilities, and communication. Key stakeholders include the CPHQ, the disaster response team, the administration, the public health department, police, first responders, and fire departments. Disasters can include a multi-casualty influx of individuals from a community emergency, such as a train accident; an epidemic; fire or other internal hospital problem requiring evacuation; or inadequate staffing to safely treat ED individuals. Plans should include/address:

- Readily available information and disaster preparedness drills.
- Activation of the plan, including the individual(s) responsible.
- Chain of command.
- Facility damage assessment, usually conducted by plant safety officer.
- Hospital/ED capacity to receive individuals.
- Triage, including in community and in the ED.
- Transfer protocols for distributing individuals to other facilities.
- Staffing, including telephone tree to notify staff to report to facility.
- Intra- and Inter-facility communication and communication with pre-hospital EMS personnel.

- Supplies on hand and methods to obtain added supplies.
- Delineation of receiving and treatment areas.

PROMOTING QUALITY AND SAFETY THROUGH CORPORATE COMPLIANCE

The Office of Inspector General of HHS issues **corporate compliance** guidance for different types of healthcare organizations. Corporate compliance requires adherence to state and federal regulations and legal and ethical standards. Because compliance issues are so broad and complex, the organization should have a compliance officer with expertise to review all compliance issues and ensure that the organization complies. Compliance issues include:

- Privacy and Security concerns of HIPAA, HITECH, including conducting audit trails.
- Accountability standards: Discipline, confidentiality, and privacy policies.
- Regulatory requirements: Include ADA, CMS, CLIA, EMTLA, OSHA, EEOC, Anti-Kickback Statute, Stark Law (limiting referrals by physicians), Fair Labor Standards Act, Family and Medical Leave Act, and Federal Wage Garnishment Law.
- Record retention policies and practices.
- Screening/Employment standards and practices, including appropriate interviewing (hiring and exit).
- Third party due diligence: Vendors, contractual agreements.
- Communication of regulatory requirements and education in compliance issues.
- Risk assessment and compliance audits (internal, external).
- Investigations and disclosures of non-compliance.
- Government sanctions lists: Including country-specific lists as well as terrorism and narcotics sanctions lists. OIG exclusions of individuals.
- Organizational transparency and culture of compliance.

PROMOTING QUALITY AND SAFETY THROUGH PROVIDER NETWORKS

Provider networks are specific types of healthcare insurance plans in which claims from healthcare providers in a network are reimbursed at a higher level than claims from healthcare providers who are outside of the network. The provider network comprises a group of healthcare providers (physicians, therapists, advance practice RNs, hospitals) who have a contractual agreement to provide services at a prescribed fee via a paid-provider organization (PPO), a health maintenance organization (HMO) or an exclusive provider organization (EPO). The board of directors and administration are often key stakeholders in utilizing a provider network rather than other types of plans because provider networks provide negotiated discounts for treatment and may also provide substantial savings in healthcare costs. However, costs may also be substantial for participants who choose an out-of-network provider, and individuals seeking care must first determine which healthcare providers are in the network. Provider networks often have preauthorization requirements, such as before expensive procedures (MRI, angiography) or surgery.

INTERDISCIPLINARY COLLABORATION

Interdisciplinary collaboration is absolutely critical to medical practice if the needs and best interests of the patients and families are central. Interdisciplinary practice begins with the nurse and physician, and extends to pharmacists, social workers, Occupational Therapists, physiotherapists, nutritionists, lab technologists, and a wide range of allied healthcare providers, all of whom cooperate in diagnosis and treatment. State regulations determine how much *autonomy* a nurse has in diagnosing, treating, and prescribing. While nurses have gained more legal rights, they have also become more dependent on collaboration with others for their expertise and for referrals, if the patient's needs extend beyond the nurse's ability to provide assistance. Some states require direct supervision of nurses by physicians, dentists, or other licensed practitioners. Other states allow indirect supervisory arrangements, depending on the circumstances. For example, nurse practitioners have much more latitude than new grads.

LINKING PATIENT SAFETY ACTIVITIES WITH STRATEGIC GOALS

Linking patient safety activities with the strategic goals of the organization is an important step in developing a plan for patient safety. The governing board and leadership must re-evaluate the strategic goals periodically, and revise them as part of the organization's commitment to safety. Strategic goals may be expressed in terms that are very broad, such as "Improve patient safety," but these **broad goals** should be coupled with more **specific objectives**, such as "Decrease post-operative infections." As part of the linkage procedure, activities must be identified that relate to each strategic goal and objective, and the data collection method and expected measurable outcomes should be specified for each activity, with a **timeline**. For example, "Decrease the number of surgical site infections by 40% by September 1." Goals for measurable outcomes should be based on **assessment** and **data**, so that they are achievable with adherence to performance improvement activities.

Consultative Support and Governing Bodies

GOVERNANCE INFRASTRUCTURE

Understanding the **governance infrastructure** of an organization is necessary for integrating quality findings. Organizations incorporated by state charter are required to have a ***governing body***, which carries legal authority and responsibility for all care provided by the organization. The governing body is organized under by-laws, in accordance with both state and federal regulations. The factors that impact the board's ability to effect change are:

- Size and structure of the board.
- Experience and knowledge of its members.
- Management infrastructure, including leadership, objectives, agendas, meetings, education, and assessment.
- Functions, roles and responsibilities, such as formulating vision and strategic goals, ensuring quality, developing policies, decision-making, and oversight.

INTEGRATING QUALITY FINDINGS

INTEGRATING QUALITY FINDINGS INTO GOVERNANCE AND MANAGEMENT ACTIVITIES

Integrating quality findings into **governance and management activities** requires a commitment from the governing board and administration to restructuring and re-engineering. Findings must be incorporated into the ***strategic goals***, and by-laws and administrative policies must be realigned to reflect a change in focus. This process requires broad changes to offer a seamless continuum of care:

- Aligning payment and incentive systems, to tie rewards to clinical objectives for improving health care.
- Establishing a new culture of organization-wide management, rather than focusing management on departments.
- Integrating the administrative and management infrastructure to include planning for resource allocation, marketing, human resource development, and quality care.
- Assessing populations to determine needs within the community.
- Providing services in accordance with needs assessment, including adequate access to services.
- Utilizing technology for assessment and evaluation.
- Establishing critical care pathways and protocols, and utilizing continuous improvement processes with interdisciplinary teams.
- Establishing case management.

INTEGRATING QUALITY FINDINGS IN BY-LAWS

The **by-laws** of the governing body define lines of authority, responsibility, accountability and communication within the organization. By-laws specify the formation and structure of the governing board, and the procedures for selecting officers and committees. The by-laws establish the relationship between the governing board and the medical staff and define conflicts of interest. By-laws specify lines of authority and responsibility at all levels in the organization related to quality, safety, patient care, credentialing, privileging, and performance improvement. Budget development and approval of the budget is a central purpose of the governing board because budget considerations directly impact quality of patient care and the ability of the organization to carry out substantial changes. As part of the budget process, the by-laws provide that the governing board plans for organization-wide services.

24

INTEGRATING QUALITY FINDINGS INTO STRATEGIC GOALS

The governing board must establish a method by which quality management activities and issues are reported to them. Once the board has established **strategic goals** based on quality findings and input from quality professionals, the board must ensure *integration* of the findings into governance and management. It must:

- Provide organization-wide support for strategic goals.
- Utilize performance improvement measures as part of business planning and resource allocation.
- Support use of performance measures to provide current information about performance organization-wide, such as with balanced scorecards or dashboards.
- Provide resources for education and training.

Participate in oversight activities through creation of oversight teams or committees, including review of summary reports regarding performance improvement activities, public reporting, and validation of compliance with licensing, credentialing, and privileging regulations or by-laws

INTEGRATING QUALITY FINDINGS INTO MANAGEMENT ROLES

Management has a critical role in integrating quality findings into their activities. Managers must consistently look toward the future of an organization, govern growth, work toward restructuring and internalizing change, managing knowledge, and integrating best practices into processes to ensure quality. Managers must:

- Exhibit a commitment to performance improvement and create a culture of quality.
- Empower staff to facilitate change.
- Provide adequate training, support, and resources for performance improvement activities.
- Participate in the quality improvement process and incorporate it into job descriptions.
- Evaluate compliance with quality performance goals.
- Monitor effectiveness of performance activities and conduct evaluations.
- Provide continuous education regarding quality performance to all levels of the organization.
- Provide reports and education to the governing board.

INTEGRATING ACCREDITATION AND REGULATORY RECOMMENDATIONS

Accreditation and regulatory recommendations should always be considered minimal, rather than optimal, standards for an organization. View the surveyors' recommendations from the perspective that the institution has failed to meet minimum standards. Use positive reports as part of rewards and positive performance appraisals. Recommendations should trigger these responses to integrate the recommendations into the organization:

- Administrative commitment to utilize resources to meet and exceed recommendations.
- Organization-wide education of standards and compliance issues.
- Root cause analysis to determine areas of improvement.
- Utilization of analysis as part of peer review and/or performance appraisal.
- Planning and development of action plans for improvement.
- Implementation of action plans.
- Ongoing assessment and modification of plans as needed to achieve target outcomes.
- Evaluation of action plans in a report to the governing board.

Data Management

EVALUATING AND DEVELOPING DATABASES

Databases are computerized file structures that contain organized and accessible stored data. Relational databases, which are built on a multiple table structure with each individual item on a table having a unique identifier, are the most common type. When building a database, one of the first steps to ensuring adequate data is to do a requirement analysis, which can involve eliciting information about data through case studies, interviews, focus groups, and observations. Identifying the types of data and the types of interaction with the data is necessary to help determine the data needed because data input must result in desired output. A database may become inflated in size because of redundancy, so eliminating redundancy is essential. The CPHQ can provide input to identify those attributes that are key to identification and those that provide information or provide both identification and information. Then, redundant identification attributes can be removed.

EVALUATING AND DEVELOPING REGISTRIES

Registries are collections of secondary data about specific patient diagnoses, treatment, procedures, and/or conditions. A healthcare organization may develop a number of different registries in order to collect data and to make the data available to researchers as well as to track follow-up care. The CPHQ often has an active role in determining which registries to compile and the case definitions for inclusion in the registry. Common registries include: cancer, trauma, congenital defects, diabetes, cardiac conditions, HIV, transplants, and immunizations. Once the registry is established and the case definition completed, the CPHQ may develop protocols for case finding and submission of data. Some registries, such as the cancer registry, are mandated by law but others are determined by institutional need. Data elements vary according to the type of registry but may include specific demographic information, diagnosis, treatment, stages (when appropriate), status codes, and functional status.

External Best Practices

EVIDENCE-BASED PRACTICE GUIDELINES (EBP)

Evidence-based practice guidelines (EBP) for such things as standing medication orders or antibiotic protocols are in common use, but decisions are often made based on studies that lack internal and/or external validity, or on expert opinion colored by personal bias, so the process of establishing evidence-based practice guidelines should be done systematically. Include those who resist the process, to facilitate the acceptance of guidelines. However, one must base decisions on solid evidence as much as possible. Simply dispensing evidence-based practice guidelines often does not change practice. Consider how the change will be **implemented.** Decide if the guidelines are mandatory for standing orders, and to what degree individual practitioners can choose other options. Guidelines that are too rigid are counter-productive. In some cases, establishing guidelines may affect cost-reimbursement from third-party payers.

To implement evidence-based practice guidelines (EBP):

- **Focus on the topic/methodology:** List possible interventions or treatments for review. Choose patient populations and settings. Determine significant outcomes. Outline search boundaries (journal titles and types of studies). Use studies published within the last five years, unless historical trends are needed.
- **Evidence review:** Review the literature. Critically analyze studies. Summarize the results, including pooled meta-analysis.
- **Expert judgment:** If review produces inadequate evidence, use recommendations from subject matter experts (SME). Acknowledge the SME's subjective evidence in the policy.
- **Policy considerations:** Weigh cost-effectiveness, access to care, insurance coverage, availability of qualified staff, and legal implications.
- **Policy:** Write a policy for the organization's P&P manual. Letter rank recommendations, so that "A" is the most highly recommended, based on the quality of supporting evidence.
- **Review:** Submit completed policy for peer review before instituting it. Keep the authorizing signatures on file. Update and renew the policy at least every two years.

CRITICAL PATHWAYS

Critical pathways are multidisciplinary care plans, which outline care steps and expected outcomes, based on the patient's specific diagnosis, procedure, or condition. Critical pathways outline goals in patient care, and the sequence and timing of interventions to achieve those goals. Critical pathways improve and standardize care, and decrease hospital stays. There are two basic types of critical pathways:

- **Guidelines:** No documentation is required to verify that the pathway has been followed. A guideline suggests how to conduct optimal patient care. The guideline is usually a flow sheet, with different *If–Then* paths to follow, depending on the patient's outcomes.
- **Integrated Care Plan:** An ICP requires dates, signatures, and documentation to show that the steps have been carried out and to indicate specific outcomes.

Write pathways based on best practices. Monitor their effectiveness regularly. Periodically evaluate their outcomes to determine if modifications are needed to reach goals.

Critical pathways are developed by multidisciplinary teams involved in direct patient care. For example, a critical pathway for hip replacements involves a rheumatologist, surgeon, anesthetist, surgical and orthopedic nurses, physiotherapist, occupational therapist, pharmacist, nutritionist,

27

and social worker. The pathway cannot require additional staffing, and must cover the entire scope of an illness in these steps:

- Select a patient group based on data analysis and observations that show:
  - A wide variance in the current treatment approach
  - An organizational priority
  - Increasing patient needs (e.g., more hip replacements because of aging Boomers)
- Create an interdisciplinary pathway development team.
- Review literature. Study best practices. Identify opportunities for quality improvement.
- Identify all categories of care (Nutrition, Pharmacy, Nursing, etc.)
- Discuss findings and reach consensus.
- Identify levels of care and number of days covered by the pathway.
- Pilot test the pathway and redesign steps as required.
- Educate staff.
- Monitor and track variances to improve the pathway.

HEALTHCARE EFFECTIVENESS DATA AND INFORMATION SET (HEDIS)

The **Healthcare Effectiveness Data and Information Set (HEDIS)** is a tool utilized by greater than 90% of health plans to measure performance of over 80 measures in 5 domains of care: effectiveness of care, access/availability of care, experience of care, utilization and risk adjusted utilization, and relative resource. Additional domains include health plan descriptive information and measures collected using electronic clinical data systems. HEDIS data are collected from health plans and physicians and compiled in databases and can be used to compare health plan performance. HEDIS is updated annually by the National Committee for Quality Assurance (NCQA) with measures added and deleted. HEDIS data collection is through surveys and insurance claims and is mandated by CMS for Medicare Advantage HMO plans and by NCQA's accreditation process. Measures may apply to commercial health plans, Medicaid, and/or Medicare as appropriate. HEDIS data may be utilized to assess external best practices and the quality of performance, set performance goals, and identify cost-effective interventions.

Lead and Facilitate Change

LEADERSHIP

CREATING STAFF COMMITMENT

Leadership must be consistent and succeeds by providing staff with direction and guidance that shows by example, explaining why things need to be done, rather than directing how this must be achieved. A good leader fosters **values** by focusing on the right way to do things, rather than on errors or poor performance. By engaging staff in all parts of the process, a leader engenders a sense of **commitment** in the staff. Commitment cannot be achieved through rules, regulation, threats, and criticism. A good leader must demonstrate integrity, welcome diversity, be open-minded, and search for competence. While a leader must have a thorough understanding of the organization/facility and its work, he or she must be able to perceive **holistically**. The leader must motivate others by providing structure, order, and able decision-making. The leader must both **learn** and **teach** in order to create positive change.

MOTIVATING STAFF

An organization's leaders must understand staff's **motivation** to increase productivity and improve performance. Leaders who use **active listening** discover the strengths of individuals and groups within their organization. Leaders who provide positive reinforcement and rewards, expect excellence, and remove barriers to employee involvement in the work process enable their employees to feel empowered, recognized and acknowledged as valuable. Leaders must base their responses on actual **assessment**, rather than preconceived ideas or biases. The four greatest motivators for employees are:

- **Autonomy**: Allowing people to use their ideas
- **Salary**: Providing adequate compensation for work done
- **Recognition**: Appreciating the efforts that employees put forth
- **Respect**: Listening to ideas

TYPES OF LEADERS

The four **types of leaders** are:

- **Charismatic:** The charismatic leader depends on personal **charm** to influence people and is very persuasive. However, charismatic leaders have limited effectiveness because they make followers of employees, and relate to one group, rather than the organization as a whole.
- **Bureaucratic:** The bureaucrat follows the organization's **rules** exactly and expects everyone else to do the same. Bureaucrats are most effective in handling cash flow or managing work in dangerous work environments. Bureaucrats may engender respect but are not conducive to change or creativity.
- **Autocratic:** The autocrat makes decisions **independently**, and strictly enforces rules. Team members often feel left out of the decision-making process and may not be supportive. Autocratic leaders are most effective in crisis situations but may have difficulty with staff commitment for routine work.
- **Consultative:** The consultant presents a decision to staff and welcomes their **input** and questions, although the original decision rarely changes. Consultative leadership is most effective when gaining the support of staff is critical to the success of proposed changes.

LEADERSHIP STYLES

The three **leadership styles** are:

- *Participatory*: A participatory style means the leader presents a potential decision and then makes the final decision based on **input** from individual employees or teams. Participatory leadership is time-consuming and may result in compromises that are not wholly satisfactory to either management or staff, but participation motivates employees, who feel their expertise is valued.
- *Democratic*: A democratic style means the leader presents a problem and asks individual employees or teams to arrive at a **solution**, although the leader usually makes the final decision. Democratic leadership may delay decision-making, but employees and teams are often more committed to the solutions because of their input.
- *Laissez-faire (free rein):* A laissez-faire style means the leader exerts indirect control, allowing employees/ teams to make decisions **independently**, with little interference. Laissez-faire may be effective leadership if the teams are highly skilled and strongly motivated, but in many cases laissez-faire leadership is the product of poor management skills and little is accomplished because of lack of direction.

PROFESSIONAL LEADERSHIP AND ACCOUNTABILITY FOR NURSING'S ROLE

Nurses, especially those in leadership positions, have a responsibility to assist others with **professional leadership and accountability** within the healthcare team and community. Collaboration requires an ongoing commitment that includes mentoring, coaching, and teaching others. Nursing must be involved in the following:

- Making decisions at all levels of an organization/facility.
- Taking an active role in strategic planning.
- Assuming responsibility for standards of nursing care.
- Assessing and selecting equipment, supplies, and electronic information systems.
- Assisting with planning for utilization of resources.
- Analyzing all decisions with respect to patient outcomes.
- Supporting staff education and development, including training for management positions, and offering opportunities to acquire continuing education hours.
- Facilitating access to research and both internal and external resources.
- Allowing staff members time to consider their place in the organization and in their own practices.

ORGANIZATIONAL CULTURE

Organizational culture comprises the attitudes, beliefs, and behaviors of those involved in the organization. The physical environment and the organizational structure strongly impact culture. Culture involves *shared assumptions* about behavior and *working together* in an organization. To facilitate change within an organization, the leader must understand its basic underlying *values* and change the organizational culture, along with changing processes and procedures.

The **four basic types of organizational cultures** are:

- *Stable learning cultures*, where people exercise skills and advance over time
- *Independent cultures*, in which people have valued skills that are easily transferable to other organizations
- *Group cultures*, in which there is strong identification and emphasis on seniority
- *Insecure cultures*, with frequent staff layoffs and reorganizations

To facilitate changes in the organizational culture, the leader must foster a commitment to excellence at all levels, create opportunities for involvement, and empower staff. Management must be flexible, encourage team building, and systems thinking across the organization.

FACILITATING CHANGE WITHIN THE HEALTHCARE SYSTEM

Facilitating change within a healthcare organization requires the creation of a ***common vision*** for care and begins with the organization creating teams to work collaboratively and focus on serving the customers. Achieving a common vision requires a true collaborative effort:

- Include all levels of staff across the organization, encompassing nursing and all other positions.
- Build consensus through discussions, in-service training, and team meetings, so diverse viewpoints converge.
- Value staff creativity and provide encouragement during the facilitation process.
- Post the common vision statement so it is accessible to all staff.
- Recognize that a common vision is an organic concept that evolves over time, requiring regular re-evaluation and changes as needed, so it continues to reflect the needs of the organization, patients, families, and staff.

BARRIERS TO SYSTEM CHANGE

Barriers to system change can arise at the individual, departmental, or administrative levels because of:

- ***Identification with role rather than purpose***: People see themselves from the perspective of their role in the system, as nurse or physician, and are not able to step outside their preconceived ideas to view situations holistically or to accept the roles of others. They may lack the ability to look at situations as human beings first and professionals second.
- ***Feelings of victimization***: People may blame the organization or the leadership for personal shortcomings, or feel that there is nothing that they can do to improve or change situations. A feeling of victimization may permeate an institution to the point that meaningful communication cannot take place, and people are closed to change.
- ***Relying on past experience***: New directions require new solutions, so being mired in the past or relying solely on past experience can prevent progress.
- ***Autocratic views***: Autocrats feel that their perceptions and practices are the only ones that are acceptable, and often have a narrow focus, so that they cannot view the system as a whole but focus on short-term outcomes. They fail to see that there are many aspects to a problem, affecting many parts of the healthcare system.
- ***Failure to adapt***: Change is difficult for many individuals and institutions, but the medical world is changing rapidly and this requires adaptability. Those who fail to adapt may feel threatened by changes and unsure of their ability to relearn new concepts, principles, and procedures.
- ***Weak consensus***: Groups that arrive at an easy or weak consensus without delving into important issues may delude themselves into believing that they have solved problems, which remain fixed and are often ignored, rather than moving forward to resolution.

FORCE FIELD ANALYSIS

Force field analysis was designed by Kurt Lewin, a social psychologist, to analyze both the driving forces and the restraining forces for change:

- **Driving forces** instigate and promote change, such as leaders, incentives, and competition.
- **Restraining forces** resist change, such as poor attitudes, hostility, inadequate equipment, or insufficient funds.

Use this force field analysis diagram to discuss variables related to a proposed change in process:

- Write the proposed change in the center column.
- Brainstorm and list driving forces and opposed restraining forces. Score the forces. (When driving and restraining forces are in balance, this is a state of equilibrium or the status quo.)
- Discuss the value of the proposed change.
- Develop a plan to diminish or eliminate restraining forces.

CRISIS MANAGEMENT

Coordinating performance improvement involves **crisis management** preparation because the public is concerned about events that affect the quality of patient care. Consider terrorist acts, epidemics, natural disasters, financial malfeasance, public relations issues, and sentinel events when planning. Crisis management requires an organization-wide commitment to preventing crises. The two elements of crisis management are:

- *Preventive*, which includes: Establishing control barriers; conducting root cause analysis; direct observation and readiness activities; preparing contingency plans; and designing processes with failure mode and effects analyses (FMEA).
- *Reactive*, which includes: Root cause analysis of observed problems; determining long-term and short-term effects; assigning staff to deal with issues; and looking for improvement opportunities.

CONFLICT RESOLUTION

Conflict is an inevitable product of teamwork. The team leader assumes responsibility for **conflict resolution** and has a plan ready. Conflicts can be disruptive, or they can produce positive outcomes by opening dialogue and allowing team members to experience different perspectives. The best time for conflict resolution is when differences first emerge, before open conflict and hardened positions appear. Use active listening. Reassure those involved that their viewpoints are understood. Follow these steps for conflict resolution:

1. Allow both sides to present their opinions. Focus on opinions, rather than on individuals.
2. Encourage cooperation through negotiation and compromise.
3. Keep discussions on track and avoid heated arguments.
4. Evaluate the need for renegotiation, a formal resolution process, or third-party arbitration.
5. Use humor and empathy to diffuse escalating tensions.
6. Summarize the issues. Outline key arguments.
7. Avoid forcing a resolution, if possible.

DEALING WITH RESISTANCE TO ORGANIZATIONAL CHANGE

Performance improvement processes cannot occur without organizational change, but **resistance to change** is common for many people who fear job loss or increased responsibilities. Staff may suffer from denial, lack understanding, or be frustrated by bureaucracy. The effective CPHQ anticipates resistance. Achieve cooperation with this approach:

- Be honest, informative, and tactful; give people thorough information about anticipated changes and how they will be affected, emphasizing positives.
- Be patient; allow people the time they need to contemplate changes and express anger or disagreement.
- Be empathetic; listen carefully to the concerns of others.
- Encourage participation; allow staff to propose methods of implementing change, so they feel a sense of ownership.
- Establish a climate in which all staff members are encouraged to identify the need for change on an ongoing basis.
- Present further ideas for change to management.

Eight Disciplines of Problem Solving (8D)

The Eight disciplines of Problem Solving (8D) were developed by the military and later refined by Ford Motor Company and Kepner-Trego. 8D helps teams to efficiently determine *root causes*. 8D is used primarily in the industrial sector to improve product and process, but it also has direct applications to process improvement in healthcare. The disciplines are:

- Create and define an interdisciplinary team of experts with time and commitment to change. Establish roles within the team, needs, and guidelines. The team chooses their leader.
- Identify and describe the problem, including the scope and whether it is a common cause or special cause condition. Begin the process of identifying and gathering data.
- Take **i**nterim **c**ontainment **a**ction (ICA, corrective actions) by insulating internal and external customers from problems and establishing criteria for decisions, while continuing to monitor results of the ICA.
- Identify and verify root causes and special cause conditions, using such methods as root-cause analysis, Five Whys, or Is–Is Not. Test each possible cause in accordance with the problem and data.
- Choose **p**ermanent **c**orrective **a**ction (PCA). Establish criteria. List possible long-term solutions and prioritize them. Set up barrier controls to prevent the problem from recurring before committing to the action. Identify any negative side effects from the action and correct them.
- Implement PCA and remove ICA while conducting performance measures, documenting changes, and evaluating effectiveness.
- Perform evaluation to prevent recurrence. Modify procedures as necessary. Carry out formal processes to institute and communicate changes in action. Institute staff training as needed.
- Recognize the team members for their contributions and disband the team.

Population Health and Quality Improvement

POPULATION HEALTH PROMOTION AND CONTINUUM OF CARE ACTIVITIES

HANDOFFS AND TRANSITIONS OF CARE

During **handoff and transitions of care**, patients are particularly at risk because critical information may be forgotten or overlooked. The CPHQ should promote the use of a systematic method of communication to be used during handoff procedures to ensure that information is organized and complete. Handoff procedures should be documented and adequate time allowed for communication, including questions from the receiving party. The SBAR (situation-background-assessment-recommendation) tool is commonly used for handoff. The primary purpose is to promote patient safety by ensuring that all pertinent information is conveyed:

- *Situation*: Name, age, MD, diagnosis.
- *Background*: Brief medical history, co-morbidities, review of lab tests, current therapy, IV's, VS, pain, special needs, educational needs, and discharge plans.
- *Assessment*: Review of systems, lines, tubes, and drains, completed tasks, needed tasks, future procedures.
- *Recommendations*: Review plan of care, medications, precautions (restraints, falls), treatments, wound care.

Organizations utilizing SBAR should have guidelines that advise staff exactly what should be covered in each element and a worksheet the providers can utilize to organize information.

HEALTH UTILIZATION

A number of different factors must be considered regarding **health utilization**:

- *Medical necessity:* Care provided to patients should be both necessary and appropriate for the patient's condition and needs.
- *Provision of care:* Treatment and care should be based on evidence-based practice to provide the most efficient, effective, and cost-effective care.
- *Time frame:* Care should be provided in a timely manner and within the timeframe of established benchmarks.
- *Regulatory requirements:* All regulatory requirements must be met in relation to both provision of care and reporting.
- *Drug utilization:* Drug use must be appropriate and outcomes monitored. Medications should be reconciled, and polypharmacy avoided when possible. Cost of drugs should be considered as part of prescription.
- *Patient safety issues:* The National Patient Safety Indicators should be monitored and the organization's score assessed with the goal of improving safety outcomes and exceeding benchmarks.
- *Patient insurance, resources:* The patient's ability to pay for care and to have necessary support should be considered as part of plan of care.

PROVIDING OUTCOME-BASED, COST-EFFECTIVE CARE

Outcome-based, cost-effective care integrates delivery of care with supporting data. different approaches for cost-containment and quality improvement strategies. It is bas identification of a problem, collection of data (evidence), evaluation, integration of both patient needs to deliver patient care, and re-evaluation of the process. Evidence-based ca requires a **process of change** in the healthcare system:

- Resources for staff, including guidelines, journals, and established protocols.
- A mission statement and goals that support evidence-based care.
- Staff input and dialog through in-service training, meetings, team building, mentoring, teaching, and role modeling.
- Allocation of resources and staff to gather and interpret data, assessing outcomes.
- Use of randomized controlled trials (RCT) to determine which approaches are best combined with systematic research and review.
- Retaining an individual assessment to determine if data applies to the unique circumstances of each patient.

IMPACT OF QUALITY INITIATIVES ON HOSPITAL REIMBURSEMENT

PAY FOR PERFORMANCE

Pay-for-performance (P4P) is a general term referring to programs that provide monetary incentives for hospitals and healthcare providers to improve the quality of care. Medicare's value-based purchasing program is an example of a P4P program, but there are also many other private and public P4P programs. Pay-for-performance programs are usually based on four types of quality measures:

- *Performance*: Based on carrying out practices demonstrated to improve health outcomes.
- *Outcomes*: Based on achieving positive outcomes (but does not always consider social or other variables that the healthcare provider cannot control).
- *Patient experience (satisfaction):* Based on patient's perceptions of care received and their satisfaction.
- *Structures/Technology:* Based on facilities and equipment used for care, and may reward some types of upgrades, such as an upgrade to an electronic health record.

VALUE-BASED CONTRACTS

Insurance companies are increasingly using **value-based contracts** with healthcare providers and pharmaceutical companies to base reimbursement on outcomes. Some or all of reimbursement may be withheld for negative outcomes, and bonuses may be paid for positive outcomes.

Regulatory, Accreditation, and External Recognition

LICENSURE

While accreditation processes are voluntary, **licensure** is mandatory, usually through the State Department of Health Services. Hospitals and laboratories must comply with state and federal laws and regulations in order to be licensed. Managed care organizations are usually licensed by other state departments, such as the **Department of Insurance**. There are a number of different types of licenses, and these vary slightly from one state to another:

- Acute medical and psychiatric hospitals
- Ambulatory surgical centers
- Skilled nursing facilities and sub-acute care centers
- Long-term care facilities
- Home health care agencies
- Hospice agencies
- Assisted living programs
- Residential programs for the behaviorally, mentally, and developmentally disabled

Organizations that use beds or staffing in non-compliant ways risk losing their licenses. Licenses specify the number of patient beds, the types of patients, and staffing provisions, which vary from state to state.

APPROPRIATE ACCREDITATION, CERTIFICATION, AND RECOGNITION OPTIONS

ACCREDITATION ASSOCIATION FOR AMBULATORY HEALTH CARE (AAAHC)

The **Accreditation Association for Ambulatory Health Care (AAAHC)** provides voluntary accreditation for a wide range of ambulatory care providers, including ambulatory surgery centers, dental group practice, diagnostic imaging centers, HMOs, podiatry practices, and women's health centers. AAAHC provides accreditation to the organization itself but also provides specialty-focused certification, such as orthopaedic certification. For accreditation, the organization must undergo self-evaluation, peer review, ongoing education, and an on-site survey by AAHC at least every 3 years.

COMMISSION ON ACCREDITATION OF REHABILITATION FACILITIES (CARF)

The **Commission on Accreditation of Rehabilitation Facilities (CARF)** provides voluntary accreditation to health and human service organizations, such as aging services, behavioral health, medical rehabilitation, opioid treatment programs, and child and youth services. Accreditation requires consultation with CARF resource specialist for assistance with preparation, self-evaluation, application, payment of a fee, and a survey by CARF surveyors. Accreditation may be provisional or for one to three years. To receive accreditation, the organization must conform to internationally accepted standards.

DNV GLOBAL (DNV GL)

DNV Global (DNV GL) is an accreditation organization that accredits hospitals, critical access hospitals, and ancillary services, such as home health, hospice, DMEPOS, pharmacy, and private duty. DNV GL also provides a number of certificates, including Managing Infection Risk, Primary Stroke Center, Comprehensive Stroke Center, Acute Stroke Ready, and Hip and Knee Replacement Program. DNV GL utilizes National Integrated Accreditation for Healthcare (NIAHO®) requirements and integrates CMS Conditions of Participation with ISO 9001 Quality Management program. Surveys are conducted annually.

INTERNATIONAL ORGANIZATION FOR STANDARDIZATION (ISO)

The **International Organization for Standardization (ISO)** publishes international standards. ISO 9000 includes standards for quality management and promotes a process approach utilizing the PDCA cycle and risk-based thinking. Standards are purchased for use by an organization. ISO 9001:2015 establishes necessary criteria for quality management with a focus on quality management principles: customer focus, leadership, engagement of people, process approach, evidence-based decision making, and relationship management.

BALDRIGE AWARD CRITERIA FOR PROCESS MANAGEMENT

The **Malcolm Baldrige National Quality Award** criteria for process management are models used to facilitate *process selection*. This award system has established standards of review for successful performance. Baldrige reviews process management related to: Work systems design; work process management and improvement; core competencies; disaster preparedness; customers' needs and expectations; decision-making; performance measures; and innovations. Baldrige also reviews the organization's performance and improvement in these areas:

- Key healthcare outcomes, including comparative data.
- Current levels and trends in patient and other customer satisfaction.
- Financial performance and market share.
- Process effectiveness outcomes.
- Leadership outcomes related to carrying out strategic plans, compliance with accreditation and regulatory bodies, and contributions to the community.

Baldrige also reviews how an organization utilizes measures to track performance and improve processes.

APPLYING FOR A MALCOLM BALDRIGE NATIONAL QUALITY AWARD

The **Malcolm Baldrige National Quality Award,** established by Congress in 1987, recognizes quality in healthcare. The Award program reviews applicants for *improvement in 9 areas*: Leadership; strategic planning; customer/market focus; measurement; analysis; knowledge management; Human Resources; process management; and results.

Organizations that are in the process of change for performance improvement may apply for the award. Even if an organization does not win, it will benefit from the comprehensive evaluation and objective external review of data that the examiners provide. Reviewers award points. 450 of 1,000 points pertain to outcomes, so the organization focuses on the most important performance measures. The application process includes a 50-page self-assessment that provides a valuable tool for the organization. Essentially, the Baldrige award process serves as an inexpensive consulting service. To fully benefit from the review, an organization must have already begun the work of performance improvement, with action plans developed and activities in place.

APPLYING FOR ANCC MAGNET STATUS

The American Nurses' Credentialing Center (ANCC) **Magnet Status Award** is given to healthcare organizations based on their quality of nursing care. An extensive self-assessment is required as part of the application process, which provides valuable information about nursing within the organization. The actual review provides feedback to facilitate change. However, many criteria must be met before an organization is eligible for a Magnet award. Review the nursing practice for compliance prior to application, because much time and effort is involved in applying for the award. Entrance criteria include:

- A chief nursing officer with a Master's degree and a minimum BS in Nursing, who participates in the highest decision-making and strategic planning bodies.
- Nursing administration uses ANA's standards.
- Protected feedback procedures, whereby nurses can express concerns without fear of retribution.
- No unfair labor practices committed involving a nurse for 3 years prior to application.
- Regulatory compliance.
- Data collection includes nurse-sensitive indicators.

NATIONAL COMMITTEE FOR QUALITY INSURANCE: PATIENTS' RIGHTS

Patients' rights are outlined in standards from the Joint Commission and National Committee for Quality Assurance. Rights include:

- Respect for personal dignity and psychosocial, spiritual, and cultural considerations.
- Responsiveness to needs related to access and pain control.
- Ability to make decisions about care without coercion, including informed consent, advance directives, and end-of-life care.
- Procedures for registering complaints or grievances.
- Protection of confidentiality and privacy.
- Freedom from abuse or neglect.
- Protection during research and information related to ethical issues of research.
- Appraisal of outcomes, including unexpected outcomes.
- Accessible information about organization, services, and practitioners.
- Appeal procedures for decisions regarding benefits and quality of care.
- Organizational codes of ethical behavior.
- Procedures for donating and procuring organs and tissue for transplants.

LIVING WILLS, DNR, AND DURABLE POWER OF ATTORNEY

In accordance with federal and state laws, patients have the right to **self-determination** in healthcare, including decisions about end-of-life care through **advance directives**, such as living wills and the right to assign a surrogate person to make decisions through a durable power of attorney. Patients should routinely be questioned about an advanced directive when they present at a healthcare organization. Patients who indicate they desire a "do not resuscitate" (DNR) order should not receive resuscitation or heroic measures for terminal illness or conditions in which meaningful recovery cannot occur. Patients and families of those with terminal illnesses should be questioned as to whether the patients are hospice patients. For those with DNR requests, or those who request no heroic measures and withdrawal of life support, staff should provide the patient with **palliative**, rather than curative measures. Palliative measures include pain control, oxygen supplements, physical comforts and emotional support to the patient and family. Treat religious traditions and beliefs about death with respect.

PROBLEM SOLVING

Problem solving in any nursing context involves arriving at a hypothesis and then testing and assessing data to determine if the hypothesis holds true. When a problem arises, take steps to resolve the immediate problem and then avoid a recurrence or worsening:

- **Define the issue:** Talk with the patient, family and staff to determine if the problem relates to a failure of communication or other issues, such as diverse culture or religion.
- **Collect data:** Interview additional staff, review documentation, and gain a variety of perspectives.
- **Identify important concepts:** Determine if there are issues related to values or beliefs.
- **Consider reasons for actions:** Determine the motivations and intentions of all parties that relate to the problem.
- **Make a decision:** Decide how to prevent a recurrence of the problem, based on advocacy and moral agency. Reach the best solution possible for the patient and family.

PATIENT ADVOCACY AND MORAL AGENCY

Use both internal and external resources for patient **advocacy and moral agency**:

- **Advocacy** is working for the best interests of the patient when an ethical issue arises, despite conflicts with personal values.
- **Agency** is openness and recognition of issues and a willingness to act.
- **Moral agency** is the ability to recognize and take action to influence the outcome of a conflict or decision.

Ethical issues are difficult to assess because of personal bias, so share concerns with internal resources and reach a consensus. Issues of concern include options for care, refusal of care, privacy rights, adequate relief of suffering, and the right to self-determination. Internal resources include the Ethics Committee and Risk Managers, who can provide guidance related to personal and institutional liability. External agencies include government agencies, such as the Public Health Department.

CREDENTIALING AND PRIVILEGING PROCESSES

Credentialing is a background check to verify a job candidate's diplomas, registrations, licenses, references, insurance, and other factors that determine his or her fitness to provide patient care, in accordance with the organization's bylaws. **Privileging** follows the credentialing process and grants the individual authority to practice within the organization. Many organizations use Internet services to verify credentials (e.g., Kroll Background America and IntelliSoft Group). The credentials committee determines what credentials are necessary for different positions, based on the following:

- Professional standards, such as those of the American Nurses Association
- Licensure
- Regulatory guidelines, such as state requirements
- Accreditation guidelines

Other considerations include best practices, economic considerations, malpractice insurance coverage, disciplinary actions, and organizational needs. Ensure a policy is in place for privileging temporary staff for special circumstances or for emergencies that follows the state's regulations.

CORE CRITERIA

There are many considerations for **credentialing and privileging**, some of which are internal organizational considerations that do not involve the quality of the applicant. However, **four primary core criteria** focus only on the applicant:

1. *Licensure* must be current through the appropriate state board, such as the state board of nursing.
2. *Education* is training and experience appropriate for the credential, and can be vocational, technical, professional, residencies, internships, fellowships, doctoral and postdoctoral programs, and board and clinical certifications.
3. *Competence* is determined by evaluations and recommendations from peers regarding clinical competency, judgment, and how the candidate applies knowledge.
4. *Performance ability*: The candidate must have demonstrated ability to perform the duties to which the credentialing/privileging applies.

GENERAL COMPETENCIES ADAPTED BY THE JOINT COMMISSION FOR CREDENTIAL AND PRIVILEGING

General competencies for practitioners in healthcare organizations have been adapted by the Joint Commission and apply to all healthcare settings. Competencies necessary for practice include:

- *Quality care*: Patient care provided must be compassionate, appropriate, effective, and must promote health, treat disease, and provide end-of-life support.
- *Medical/clinical knowledge*: The applicant demonstrates knowledge of current and evolving medical, social, and clinical sciences, is able to apply this to patient care, and can use this knowledge to educate others.
- *Learning*: Practice-based learning skills, based on scientific methods, should be used to improve patient care.
- *Interpersonal and communication skills*: The applicant uses interpersonal and communication skills to establish and maintain professional relationships with others.
- *Professionalism*: Applicant demonstrates commitment to professional development, ethical practice, and sensitivity to diversity.
- *Knowledge of systems*: The applicant understands all aspects of a system and can use knowledge to improve health care.

VOLUNTARY ACCREDITATION PROCESSES

Accreditation is a primary requirement for most healthcare organizations, because it establishes a commitment to standards based on evaluation. General accreditation is either done by:

- The **Joint Commission** accredits more than 20,000 healthcare programs, both nationally and internationally. It is the primary accrediting agency in the United States, so accreditation by the Joint Commission indicates a commitment to improving care and provides information about compliance with core measures.
- The **Healthcare Facilities Accreditation Program of the American Osteopathic Association**, which also accredits many healthcare programs, including acute care, ambulatory care, rehabilitation centers and substance abuse centers, behavioral care centers, and critical access hospitals. It provides guidelines for patient safety initiatives, and reports common deficiencies.

A healthcare organization may also seek accreditation by agencies with a narrower focus to demonstrate excellence in a **particular area**, such as the Intersocietal Commission for the

Accreditation of Echocardiography Laboratories (ICAEL). Leadership must determine what type of accreditation is most appropriate, based on the programs they offer and their commitment to improvement.

OBTAINING ACCREDITATION

An institution performs a **self-assessment** to ensure it complies with **standards** related to patient care, safety issues, and performance-based **core measures** (comparative measurements).

Surveyors perform a **peer review** to assess **compliance**. They scrutinize:

- Documents (e.g., policies & procedures manuals).
- Medical records.
- Standards implementation measures.
- Integration of performance measurement data.
- Service and support systems.
- Surveyors visit the institution for an **accreditation evaluation**. They inspect, observe, and interview staff in person.

The surveyors release their final **report**, which may:

- Renew an accreditation.
- Make a Conditional Accreditation (CA) or Preliminary Denial of Accreditation (PDA) if there are infractions.
- Make a Denial of Accreditation (DA) if circumstances pose a threat to staff, the public, or patients.

The institution may appeal for **reconsideration** of the surveyors' adverse decision within 60 days. Surveyors conduct a second visit for CA institutions to ensure that infractions are corrected. If appeal is denied, the institution can request a formal hearing by the FDA to demonstrate its compliance through documentation or interviews.

CPHQ'S ROLE IN ACCREDITATION AND LICENSURE

To obtain **accreditation and licensure**, a facility must meet standards set by all its regulatory agencies. For example, the Joint Commission evaluates infection control, visiting rules, patient rights, background checks, educational programs, staffing levels, medical records, and ventilation for accreditation. The guidelines by which hospitals are evaluated are very specific, such as the exact minutes after admission for pneumonia that a patient receives an antibiotic, with scores according to the elapsed time. The CPHQ reviews, understands, communicates, and establishes guidelines for all accreditation requirements to ensure all staff and departments are aware of the requirements and document compliance. The *accreditation surveyor* uses tracer methodology to evaluate the processes that are in place, so complete extensive staff training at all levels regarding processes. Use tracer methodology as part of the general assessment, so staff can practice gathering the type of information they need to supply to the accreditation surveyors.

Evaluating Compliance

JOINT COMMISSION CORE MEASURES

The Joint Commission has established **core measures** to determine if healthcare institutions are in compliance with current standards. The core measures involve a series of questions that are answered either "yes" or "no" to indicate if an action was completed. Currently, the Joint Commission's core measures are as follows:

- Acute Myocardial Infarction (AMI)
- Children's Asthma Care
- Emergency Department
- Hospital Outpatient Department
- Hospital-Based Inpatient Psychiatric Services
- Immunization
- Perinatal Care
- Stroke
- Substance Use
- Tobacco Treatment
- Venous thromboembolism

For each condition, questions relate to whether or not **standard care** was provided, such as giving an Aspirin for those patients with an acute MI. This data is public and provides useful information about these particular standards, but does not necessarily reflect the overall quality of care. Core measurements alone are not adequate performance measures, but must be considered along with other indicators.

UTILIZATION REVIEWS

A **utilization review** (UR) determines if care is medically necessary from the time of admission, treatment, and discharge, and if it adhered to critical pathways. UR evaluates whether decision-making, care, and length of the hospital stay are appropriate. ***Third-party payers*** and ***insurance companies*** conduct utilization reviews. Issues considered during UR include the severity of illness based on symptoms, history, and laboratory testing, and the intensity of service, based on diagnostic procedures and treatments. UR may result in legal actions with individual practitioners, such as intervening in care. Appeal processes for those denied coverage for treatments or care must be written and available. Appeals are considered first by an independent reviewer, and if a denial is received, a second review is conducted by independent external reviewers. States have specific regulations dealing with the appeal process.

CASE MANAGEMENT

Case management is an important tool for integrating the outcome of utilization management assessment into the performance improvement process. Utilization review and management are primarily used to determine cost effectiveness and to contain costs, but that must be balanced by individual patients' needs. The governing board and medical directors of the hospital must determine the criteria for appropriate care, based on the mission and strategic goals of the organization. The case manager screens patients from the time of admission (or before admission in some cases) and assists with discharge planning. In some cases, criteria require that second opinions be rendered before non-emergent surgery. Case managers are involved in all aspects of patient care, across disciplines:

- Assessing the plan of care.
- Coordinating treatment and providing continuity.
- Providing continuous assessment by evaluating variances to critical pathways.
- Completing evaluation and discharge planning.
- Performing a post-discharge assessment.

Three **models for case management** that can be used to integrate the outcome of utilization management assessment into the performance improvement process are:

- ***Type of provider care***: Includes self-care by the patient, primary care (patient and primary care physician), episodic care (patient, primary care physician, specialist, and case manager), and brokered care (involves community, government, or private services).
- ***Focus of care***: The focus may be on cost containment, common to managed care programs, where service depends on the program's benefits and criteria for medical necessity, and there is little or no direct contact with the patient or family. The focus may also be on coordination of care, which involves direct patient and family contact, and individualized assessment and intervention.
- ***Professional discipline***: Case management may be done by nurses, social workers, psychiatrists, or other specific disciplines, depending on the goals of case management.

INTEGRATING THE OUTCOME OF UTILIZATION MANAGEMENT ASSESSMENT

INTEGRATING INTO THE PERFORMANCE IMPROVEMENT PROCESS

The **utilization management assessment** measures and assesses the use of services, procedures, and facilities in terms of medical necessity and appropriateness. Analyze these trends:

- ***Overutilization***: Inappropriate admissions, levels of care, length of stay, or undocumented rationale for resource use (such as frequent, expensive lab tests).
- ***Underutilization***: Level of care or resources was inadequate for medical necessity (failure to admit, inadequate lab testing).
- ***Misutilization***: Errors were made in treatment, or inefficiencies occurred in scheduling.

Integrating the outcomes of utilization assessment requires intervention strategies, assessment of cost-effectiveness related to quality and risk, consideration of the need to modify the preauthorization process, peer review, and establishment of teams for process improvement.

INTEGRATING INTO QUALITY MANAGEMENT

Utilization management (UM) is an important part of assessing and resolving problems through quality management.

UM FUNCTIONS UNDER QUALITY MANAGEMENT:

- Concurrent assessment of important aspects of patient care.
- Case management to ensure resources are utilized appropriately in-patient care.
- Team assessment and review of processes to ensure they are cost-effective and maintain the quality of care.

- Identification of patterns and trends across the organization.
- Practitioner profiling, credentialing, privileging, and reprivileging includes coordinated information from all areas of review to provide an objective assessment.

PROBLEMS WITH UM HINDERING INTEGRATION OF OUTCOMES:

- Lack of coordination that interferes with the flow of information.
- Medical errors.
- Fear of malpractice driving unnecessary testing and utilization of resources.
- Lack of cost-knowledge on part of staff.
- Capitation pressure to underutilize.
- Lack of adequate community services.
- Inadequate data collection.

PATIENT FLOW MANAGEMENT

Patient flow management incorporates the outcome of utilization management assessment as it relates to the functions and processes of the organization that impact the quality of patient care. Patient flow management assesses the way the patient *moves through the system*, from triage, admission, to access of services, and discharge. Flow includes scheduling concerns and methods of routing patients through services. Departments are interdependent on each other. Only organization-wide utilization management is in the position to evaluate and integrate information and services. For example, Admissions depends on Discharges, which depends on completed imaging or laboratory studies, which in turn depend on transmission of orders and Patient Transport. Determining where the patient flow processes can be improved and where resources are underutilized, overutilized, or misutilized can drive change that effectively improves patient flow.

PROCESS VARIANCE MONITORING

Process variance monitoring is a review that uses critical pathways as a basis for processes involved in medical care. A **variance** is a deviation from the pathway. The variance may result from a part of the process not being performed or from the process not resulting in anticipated outcomes. Process variance monitoring creates a large amount of data. It is most effective when it is targeted to critical outcomes, where variance negatively impacts patients. Document variances and take corrective steps as necessary. If the purpose is to modify or improve a pathway, variance data should be computerized and aggregated. Process variance monitoring is not used to identify individuals who are at fault, but rather to identify faulty processes.

Medication Usage Review

MEDICAL REVIEW PROCESS

Medical review processes are mandated by regulations and accreditation. Types include:

- **Prospective reviews** include all those steps taken before an event, such as assessing need before care, checking credentials before hiring, determining ability to pay prior to doing elective procedures, and gaining preauthorization from insurance companies.
- **Concurrent reviews** include ongoing assessment while the patient is receiving care, verification of medical necessity for continued treatment, and appropriate use of resources. Concurrent review uses medical records, observations of care, incidence reports, and special case studies.
- **Retrospective reviews** are conducted after care is completed and provides a full picture of the continuum of care and its effectiveness. Medical records and the results of prospective and concurrent reviews are used.
- **Focused reviews** include reviews done for specific, predetermined reasons, such as a particular diagnosis, procedure, or process. Criteria for case selection must be clearly outlined.

Develop a flow chart for a **medication usage review**, which lists all steps in the process of medication use and the disciplines involved. This overview is necessary before a more targeted review can be accomplished:

- Process Review
- Selecting medications
- Purchase order for supplier
- Receiving
- Storage
- Prescribing
- Transcribing orders
- Ordering from Pharmacy
- In-patient unit receiving from Pharmacy
- Scanning barcodes
- Preparing and dispensing
- Recording in the computer or patient's chart
- Administration
- Monitoring patient's response to medication

PURPOSE OF A MEDICATION USAGE REVIEW

The physician and pharmacist determine the **purpose** and **scope** of a medication review, and methods of data collection. **Medication usage reviews** are conducted with different parameters, depending on their purpose:

- Determine compliance with accreditation standards.
- Evaluate potential cost savings.
- Study the correlation of drugs with outcomes to improve patient care.
- Evaluate staff education related to best practices.

- To detect medication errors, observe error patterns, determine methods to avoid errors, and chart adverse reactions.
- Determine if critical pathways have been followed, and to develop further critical pathways or modify existing ones.

SCOPE AND DATA COLLECTION

The **scope of a medication review** directly relates to its purpose. The scope of the review can be:

- Very broad, including quantifying all prescriptions for medications within an organization.
- Narrowed to those patients and staff in one area or department.
- Focused on individual use of prescribed medications.
- Include or exclude outpatient prescriptions.
- Include all classes of medications, or focus on one or more, such as antibiotics.
- Examine the difference in generic and brand name drug use.

Review current tracking methods for adequacy of data collection. Paper data collection is extremely time-consuming. If prescriptions and medication dispensing are computerized, then measurements are more accurate and easier to obtain. Consider bar coding, unit dose packaging, automated drug dispensing machines (ADDM) and a computerized recording system that links the Lab, nursing unit, and Pharmacy.

SYSTEMATIC APPROACH TO MEDICAL RECORD REVIEWS

A **systematic approach to medical record reviews** requires planning and consistency. Surveillance may involve:

- ***Targeted medical record review*** with reporting forms that include all necessary information in one form, paper or electronic.
- ***Standardized questionnaires*** designed to obtain quantifiable information, featuring clear, unambiguous, and non-threatening questions. Open-ended questions may be appropriate for some types of information gathering, especially in relation to information that may be embarrassing or identifies staff errors.
- ***Consistent coding*** of data collection, with specific codes for units, populations, and individuals to facilitate analysis. Thus, the report of a patient with a cough has the same identification code as the laboratory work for that patient.
- ***Electronic surveillance*** triggered by threshold data. Reports are directly integrated with the data analysis system.

Infection Control Surveillance

SURVEILLANCE PLANS

The **purpose of a surveillance plan** is clearly outlined by the CPHQ and Infection Control Manager. Include the following elements:

- Identify a means to decrease nosocomial infections.
- Evaluate the effectiveness of infection control measures.
- Establish endemic threshold rates and enact control measures to reduce rates.
- About 5–10% of infections occur in outbreaks, so, if the CPHQ analyzes data analysis in a regular and timely manner, it establishes if the disease is endemic or an outbreak.
- Convince staff to cooperate with infection control measures by presenting objective evidence.
- Report infection rates to Public Health, the CDC, and those accreditation agencies that require reports.
- Provide a defense for malpractice suits and decrease liability by accumulating evidence that the facility is proactive in combating infections.
- Compare the facility's infection rates with similar facilities', to focus attention and resources.

INFECTION CONTROL SURVEILLANCE PLAN

The **steps in an infection control surveillance program** are:

1. Establish the parameters and design of the survey by determining what will be surveyed, when, and how, with clear definitions to guide the process.
2. Data collection must be consistent, efficient, and accurate, whether manual or automated. Sources include laboratory reports, medical records of targeted patients, interviews, and autopsy reports.
3. Data summary must make information easily accessible and available for further analysis.
4. Data analysis uses statistical measurements appropriate to the data and goals. Frequency of analysis varies but must ensure adequate numbers for the results to be meaningful.
5. Analytical interpretation involves using data to indicate threshold rates, clusters, outbreaks, and adverse events.
6. Results of analytical interpretation must be used to ameliorate the event. For example, if a threshold for infections is exceeded, clearly define procedures for dealing with that event.

ACTIVE AND PASSIVE SURVEILLANCE PLANS

Active surveillance is a program specifically designed for finding nosocomial infections, using trained and certificated staff, such as Infection Control nurses. Active surveillance is more accurate than passive surveillance because its data is more complete and consistent, since it comes from an established program. However, active surveillance is also expensive because it requires dedicated staff.

Passive surveillance uses observations from medical and laboratory staff to identify and report infections, often requiring the staff to fill out a report and submit it. Passive surveillance often results in misclassification, delays, or failure to report infections because no one is specifically charged with reporting. Staff involved in patient care may not have time to fill out reports.

PATIENT-BASED AND LABORATORY-BASED SURVEILLANCE PLANS

Patient-based surveillance plans revolve around the patient, so the patient must be assessed for signs of infection, risk factors, quality of patient care, and staff compliance with infection control protocols. Patient-based plans are very time and staff intensive, requiring much time on the in-patient units to review charts, assess patients, and interview patients and staff. For large facilities, the cost of effective patient-based plans is prohibitive.

Laboratory-based plans depend on reviews of laboratory findings, usually cultures, to determine if threshold rates are exceeded. Laboratory findings are usually accurate, but the effectiveness of this type of plan depends on completeness of records and whether specimens are correctly collected and sent to the laboratory for analysis. If there are no clear protocols in place to determine when a specimen should be obtained, infections are missed. Lab plans have electronic monitoring systems, saving staff time.

PROSPECTIVE AND RETROSPECTIVE SURVEILLANCE PLANS

Prospective, or concurrent, surveillance follows patients while they are hospitalized and includes the 30-day period after discharge to evaluate for surgical site infections. Because prospective surveillance is ongoing and continually evaluated, it identifies clusters of infection as they occur, ensuring that Infection Control personnel have ongoing working relationships with other staff. When there appears to be an outbreak or cause for concern, analysis can be done fairly quickly.

Retrospective surveillance is conducted after the fact by a review of charts and records, with no patient contact. There is a delay between the time a problem presents and the time it is identified. Retrospective surveillance is less expensive because it is ad hoc.

PRIORITY-DIRECTED AND POST-DISCHARGE SURVEILLANCE

Priority-directed surveillance is also called surveillance by objective. It ranks infection surveillance efforts in order of their importance for meeting particular goals. Serious infections are identified based on morbidity and mortality rates, costs, and the effectiveness of preventive measures based on the data. Therefore, priority-directed surveillance is often directed at surgical site infections and pneumonia. Other infections are not simply ignored, but most resources are expended in focused areas.

Post-discharge surveillance is not standardized, so it misses up to 50% of surgical site infections in patients who have short hospital stays. Patients are contacted directly through mailed questionnaires or by telephone. Sometimes, physicians are contacted for information. Readmission data is evaluated, and in some cases, patients are followed in clinics or office visits. Data is often insufficient because of difficult follow-up.

LIMITATIONS OF TARGETED SURVEILLANCE VS. HOSPITAL-WIDE SURVEILLANCE

The major **problem with hospital-wide surveillance** is its prohibitive costs in time and money. However, hospital-wide surveillance is necessary to detect all infections and to get a clear idea of the infection control problems at a facility. When the CDC National Nosocomial Infections Surveillance system (NNIS) was in place (1992-2004), it required hospital-wide surveillance, but discontinued this in favor of targeted surveillance in 1999 because most hospitals could not afford comprehensive surveillance. Infection Control still does some hospital-wide surveillance because only about 20% of hospital-acquired infections occur in the ICU, the main targeted area. Only about 19% of hospital-acquired infections involve surgical sites. Use an electronic monitoring program that automatically flags suspicious lab results, such as TheraDoc or STELLARA™. Create a rotating system for monitoring different units for specified periods of time to gain a more comprehensive picture of infections.

PRE-DESIGNED SURVEILLANCE SOFTWARE

Managing data manually is unwieldy. Use standard spreadsheet software that is packaged with most computers for simple reporting and database functions (e.g., Excel and Access). Multiple variables are more difficult to manage on a spreadsheet, and require extensive customization. Use **pre-designed surveillance software** packages to save time and expense, and yield more accurate data. Statistical packages, like SAS, SPSS, and MINITAB, have a steep learning curve. The CDC provides a free program, **Epi Info,** which was originally designed for outbreak investigation, but can manage and analyze data. It consists of these programs:

- Nutstat (a nutritional program)
- MakeView (to design data entry screens)
- Enter (to enter data into screens designed with MakeView)
- Epi Map (to link data to maps)
- Data Compare and Epi Report (for various types of statistical analysis)
- Epi Lock for privacy and data compression

POPULATION ASSESSMENT

Assessment of population is a very important component of a surveillance plan because each facility deals with a unique population. *Population* refers to that segment of patients who will be studied, because studying all patients, especially in large facilities, is impractical. Assessing a population leads to targeted surveillance where particular areas, procedures, or types of patients are surveyed. Assessment means identifying:

- Types of patients for evaluation, including medical and surgical, and frequent diagnoses.
- Commonly performed procedures and treatments, especially those that are invasive.
- Liability issues in relation to those patients that affect liability and costs.
- Community health issues, such as outbreaks, to target populations.
- Risk factors for infection as part of needs assessment.
- Facility resources and support because staff assistance is critical.

JOINT COMMISSION'S ROLE IN THE DEVELOPMENT OF INFECTION CONTROL PROGRAMS

The Joint Commission accredits most healthcare facilities in the United States. It established a requirement in 1969 that hospitals have both committees for infection control and isolation facilities in response to a growing concern about hospital-acquired infections. The Joint Commission plans to "reduce the risk of health care-associated infections" to both patients and health care workers. The Joint Commission lists extensive **standards** for surveillance, prevention, and control of infection with which healthcare facilities must comply. These guidelines and an organized infection control program are explicit accreditation requirements. Many healthcare facilities incorporate Joint Commission wording regarding infections into their infection control mission statement. Hospitals are given an accreditation report that is publicly listed, showing their compliance with goals established by the Joint Commission. **Joint Commission International** accredits hospitals throughout the world.

NOSOCOMIAL INFECTIONS

Nosocomial infection is defined by the National Healthcare Safety Network (NHSN) as a hospital-acquired infection, either localized or systemic, caused by a pathogen or toxin that was not present (or incubating) in the patient at the time he or she entered the hospital. Some infections are obvious within the first 24–48 hours, but other infections may not be obvious until after discharge from the hospital because incubation times and resistance varies. An infection that occurs within **30 days after discharge,** but is **hospital-acquired,** is nosocomial. Nosocomial infections are identified from analysis of laboratory results and clinical signs and symptoms. A diagnosis of infection by an attending physician or surgeon is also considered acceptable identification. Placentally-transferred infections are not considered nosocomial, but perinatal infections are, even if acquired from the mother during delivery. Colonization that is not causing an inflammatory response or evidence of infection is not considered nosocomial for reporting purposes.

DETERMINING THE INCIDENCE OF NOSOCOMIAL INFECTIONS

The **incidence of nosocomial specific time period infections** is the number of **new occurrences** of infections (numerator data) in a **population at risk** (denominator data) during a time that is the same for both numerator and denominator. The **incidence rate** is the number of events (numerator) divided by the number of the population at risk (denominator), often expressed as the number of infections per 100 patients. Incidence may also be used to calculate **incidence density**, which is the rate at which disease occurs in relation to the size of the population without disease. Incidence density uses the number of infections (numerator) in relation to units of time (denominator), such as the number of infections that occur in 1,000 patient days. Incidence may also be used to calculate **attack rate,** expressed as a percentage of a population at risk (denominator data) over a given time period.

CDC DEFINITIONS FOR NOSOCOMIAL INFECTIONS

In 1988, the Centers for Disease Control established the *CDC Definitions for Nosocomial Infections* to standardize reporting and obtain meaningful data for a national database. Definitions include:

- **Infection site:** For example, a urinary tract infection is coded as UTI and a surgical site infection is coded as SSI.
- **Code:** The site of infection is further coded according to the sub-type: SUTI, systematic urinary tract infection: ASB, asymptomatic bacteriuria; and OUTI, other infections of the urinary tract.
- **Definition:** The definition of the infection outlines the criteria for inclusion into a coded category. For example, UTI-SUTI (urinary tract infection–systematic urinary tract infection) includes 4 different criteria. For example, Criterion 1 is defined as:
  - Patient has at least 1 of the following signs or symptoms with no other recognized cause: Fever (>38°C), urgency, frequency, dysuria, or suprapubic tenderness AND patient has a positive urine culture, that is $\geq 10^5$ microorganisms per cm^3 of urine with no more than 2 species of microorganisms.

USING STANDARDIZED DEFINITIONS

For internal or external comparison data to be valid there must be **consistency in definitions** as to what comprises a nosocomial infection, including onset, symptoms, and laboratory findings. Clear definitions must be in place for events, indicators, and outcomes.

Events are usually defined according to the CDC definitions for nosocomial infections, but if the institution has other definitions they must be used consistently and cannot then be compared to events using other definitions.

Indicators are a measure of quality because they represent numerator data (the number of events that are being targeted, such as specific types of infections, defined as narrowly as possible). The denominator data is the population at risk for the indicator event.

Outcomes are measurements of indicators, such as the number of infections per a specified denominator, such as 100 patient days, or 1,000 device days. Outcomes should provide feedback.

NATIONAL NOSOCOMIAL INFECTIONS SURVEILLANCE (NNIS)

In 1970, the National Centers for Infectious Diseases of the U.S. Centers for Disease Control and Prevention (CDC) established the **National Nosocomial Infections Surveillance (NNIS)** system. The purposes were to encourage hospitals to report and track nosocomial infections, to use standardized methods to collect and analyze data, and to create a national database. About 300 hospitals, whose identity remained confidential, reported data using "surveillance components" and protocols that had been standardized and used CDC definitions. Surveillance components included:

- Adult and pediatric Intensive Care Units (ICUs)
- High-risk nurseries (HRN)
- Surgical patients
- Antimicrobial use and resistance

All ICU and HRN patients were surveyed, but hospitals chose from a list of surgical procedures those that they wanted to monitor for surgical patients, as the numbers of procedures done at different hospitals vary widely. Infection statistics were compiled and reported every 3 years. In 2004 this system was absorbed into the National Healthcare Safety Network (NHSN), now responsible for conducting and generating surveillance reports on nosocomial infections.

Service Quality

CUSTOMERS

A **customer** is a receiver.

Internal customers are those directly involved in product or healthcare delivery, such as the Board of Directors, administrators, clerical staff, nurses, medical support staff, physicians, Human Resources personnel, plant managers, pharmacists, and volunteer staff. Internal customers need others in the work environment to provide some type of product or service in order for them to function, and they, in turn, provide a product or service to others, so each internal customer is also a *supplier*.

Vertical customer/supplier relationships, such as between administration and nursing staff, are sometimes more obvious than the equally important *horizontal relationships*, such as between floor nurses, which involve cooperative measures to ensure that quality care is provided. Identify these types of customer/supplier relationships in the strategic plan to help increase internal awareness and improve methods of meeting the various customers' needs.

External customer-supplier relationships are critical to an organization because these customers are those that receive products or services supplied by the organization's workers. *External customers* include patients and their families, private physicians, vendors, insurance companies, government regulatory agencies, lawyers, and others in the community. As with internal customers, each external customer is both a *receiver* of products or services and a *supplier*. For example, a regulatory agency provides regulations and guidelines as a supplier, and then receives reports in return as a customer. This symbiotic relationship must be clearly understood by the CPHQ, because the external customer-supplier relationship is one over which the organization often has less direct control, so identification of the customers' needs through surveys, interviews, focus groups, research, and brainstorming can help to clarify and improve these relationships.

ASSESSING CUSTOMER NEEDS

Teams can assess customer needs as both providers and customers, so their perspective is different than that of focus groups. Teams should be interdisciplinary. Members should represent all the different *steps* in a process, in order to better understand the needs of the customers. Because team members are actively involved in the process and share objectives, even though their individual responsibilities differ, they are concerned for the customers and can generate ideas about change and reach consensus from a solid knowledge base. Teams meet and discuss issues related to customer needs, identifying customers, sharing perspectives, and generating lists of recommendations for process improvement. A *team leader* is responsible for keeping members focused on task, and ensures that all members participate, rather than one or two dominating the meetings. The team leader is also responsible for summarizing and reporting findings related to assessment.

Surveys are valuable tools to assess both customer needs and improvement progress. Take care with the survey design, because it must have validity. Before beginning, decide on these variables:

- *Target group*: Who will receive the survey? Do you need an entire population of customers (e.g., all discharge patients), or only a percentage (e.g., 30% of discharges from the Emergency Department), or some other sampling? Identifying the target group can be complex.

- **_Type of survey_:** There are different investments of time and money for paper, telephone, and Internet surveys, so check the budget.
- **_Type of questions_:** Questions with a yes/no decision are usually easier to quantify than open-ended questions or scales, although scales are frequently used to assess the degree of satisfaction.
- **_Format_:** Do font size, color, and general layout comply with the _Americans with Disabilities Act_?
- **_Follow-up:_** Survey completion rates are often low. Think up incentives for people to complete surveys. Prepare reminder letters if receiving a low response.

Practitioner Performance Evaluation

EVALUATING COMPLIANCE AND DOCUMENTATION FOR REGULATORY AND ACCREDITATION EFFORTS

The CPHQ must update **documentation** requirements based on changes to regulatory or accreditation standards. This means that the CPHQ must be cognizant of accreditation standards, such as those by the Joint Commission, and current regulations, such as those related to CMS or HIPAA, and monitor closely to determine if current documentation is adequate or if changes must be made. Accreditation standards require huge amounts of paperwork to demonstrate compliance, so building requirements into the system can save time when reports are due; thus, the CPHQ must consider the need to retrieve data as well as document necessary information when updating. While CMS provides updates regarding most federal regulations, states may have additional requirements that must be accommodated. Changes should be done well in advance of required compliance so that staff members can become familiar with changes and problems with changes can be evaluated.

PEER REVIEW

JOINT COMMISSION'S FOCUS ON PEER REVIEW

Peer review is an examination of one practitioner by a like practitioner who has similar training, experience, and expertise. If the pool of practitioners is too small within an organization, arrange an external peer review. Peer review is often triggered by root cause analysis that indicates the need to focus on an individual, sometimes related to utilization review. The Joint Commission focuses on the process of peer review in both design and function:

The **design** includes:

- A definition of a peer
- The method for selecting the peer review panel
- Triggering events
- Timeframes
- An outline of how the person being reviewed participates
- Decisions based on solid reason and literature review

The **function** is:

- Consistently applied to all individuals
- Balanced and fair
- Adherent to timelines
- Ongoing
- Valuable to the organization
- Defensible

PARTICIPATION IN PEER REVIEW

Peer review is an intensive process in which an individual practitioner is reviewed by like practitioners. Peer review can examine the practitioner's work with an individual patient or a group of patients, and often relates to data found as part of root cause analysis, infection control, or other surveillance measures. A ranking system indicates **compliance** with standards:

- Care is based on standards and is typical of that provided by like practitioners.
- Variance in care occurs, but outcomes are satisfactory.
- Care is inconsistent with that provided by like practitioners.
- Variance resulted in negative outcomes.
- In some cases, this ranking system is replaced with a series of questions, with affirmative answers indicating cause for concern.

IMPACT OF THE HEALTHCARE QUALITY IMPROVEMENT ACT (HCQI) ON PEER REVIEW

Congress passed the **HCQI of 1986** to ensure the quality of medical care by reviews, and to discipline physicians providing poor quality care or who engage in unprofessional conduct. HCQI confers limited immunity on those engaged in the peer review process if they follow the procedural provisions of the Act to ensure fairness. HCQI created the **National Practitioner Data Bank**, so that incompetent individuals must be reported, preventing them from simply moving practice to another state, and requiring organizations to request information about physicians applying for work. Prior to the passage of HCQI, physicians involved in peer review were subject to antitrust lawsuits for using the process to decrease competition. Practitioners are evaluated by **peer review** when:

- They apply for membership or reappointment.
- Root cause analysis or complaints about an individual physician set off a trigger.
- The potential for abuse exists in peer review, so ensure organization rigorously follows federal and state regulations.

PRACTITIONER PROFILING

Practitioner profiling provides practitioner-specific data and an information summary as part of reappraisal for recredentialing or reprivileging. Ideally, this is an ongoing process, or is performed every 1–2 years, as required for *credentialing*. Profiling documents both areas of concern and positive outcomes, must remain confidential, and is released only according to the bylaws of the organization and for peer review. Reviews must be signed by appropriate management/supervisory staff, such as medical directors. Profiles should include the following information:

- Clinical monitoring, including mortality rates and peer-reviewed events with negative ratings.
- Practices placing patients at risk, including operative procedures, medications, and blood product administration.
- Healthcare-related infection rates.
- Utilization management findings, including readmissions and average length of stay (ALOS).
- Patient safety findings related to root cause analysis.
- Findings of Risk Management and medical record reviews.

EMPLOYEE PERFORMANCE APPRAISAL SYSTEM

Performance appraisal is a supervisory function used to confirm hiring, promote, train, or reward staff. It should be performed when the employee's probationary period ends and on an annual basis thereafter. Supervisors who perform the appraisal should use objective data and standards, and should know and have observed the employee who is being appraised. Review the employee's *job description* first, which includes expectations and goals related to performance. Indicate in the written appraisal if the employee complies with performance expectations. Determine the role the employee has in processes and incorporate findings from performance improvement measures in the evaluation. The appraisal form may include a rating scale, checklist, productivity studies, and narrative. Discuss the appraisal with the employee, so he or she has an opportunity to respond. The employee must establish **new goals**, based on findings from performance improvement measures and related to strategic plans of the organization.

INCORPORATING FINDINGS FROM PERFORMANCE IMPROVEMENT

Findings from performance improvement are increasingly part of **credentialing, appointments, and privileging delineation,** as clinical guidelines and accountability have become accepted medical practice. Consider how the individual practitioner adheres to standards. Clinical privileges are delineated based on criteria established by the organization, and are specific to the practitioner's area of expertise. Privilege control sheets outline the level of competency necessary for each privilege granted. Competency levels are based on best practices and performance improvement data. Privileges are granted for a specific period of time, and not for the lifetime of the practitioner. The Joint Commission sets continuing education requirements for accreditation and demands documented completion of continuing education courses for credentialing.

Patient Experience Reviews

Focus Groups

Focus groups are valuable tools for assessing customer needs. Choose 8–12 participants who *share characteristics* with the group that needs to be research (e.g., age, ethnic background, community affiliation, health history, healthcare providers). Arrange for the group to meet for 1.5–2 hours for a focused discussion on a particular topic. Identify a facilitator or moderator and a recorder. It may be beneficial to observe from behind a one-way mirror, such as those found in psychiatric interview rooms. *Non-traditional focus groups* are sometimes conducted by conference telephone calls, Internet groups, or videoconferences. Focus groups are told the topic before the discussion, and often begin by sharing stories. For example, if emergency care is the focus, then all participants tell about their experiences in an Emergency Department. Then, the *facilitator* asks the group to focus on a few aspects of some stories in detail. The stories are retold, and the facilitator asks questions to obtain more details. The facilitator asks the group to respond to the stories with their reactions, comments, and questions. The *recorder* prepares a transcript of the meeting for study.

Using Traditional Focus Groups to Assess Customer Needs and Expectations

The advantages of using traditional **focus groups**, rather than electronic groups, to assess customer needs and expectations are:

- The facilitator guides the discussion to ensure that topics of interest are covered adequately, and that all members participate, keeping the discussion focused on the topic.
- The focus can be modified as needed, to allow for discussion of new ideas.
- The non-confrontational method of allowing people to share experiences allows for expression of new ideas.
- Administration or researchers may observe the interactions through the one-way mirror and communicate with the facilitator regarding further questions.
- The participants are fully involved in the process.
- Non-verbal behavior, such as facial expressions and gestures, can be observed.
- Participants are pre-screened and identified prior to the focus group meeting, and participants are not influenced by others outside the group, as may occur with telephone or Internet focus groups.

Pathology Reviews

Pathology services are of critical importance to the healthcare organization because the majority of healthcare decisions for most patients are based on clinical pathology. Review topics of particular concern to pathology include:

- *Technology*: Outline the degree and type of automated testing, computerized reporting, and linkage to all departments within the organization
- *Patient safety*: Describe monitoring, supervision, adequate staffing, consistent practices to ensure quality, and use of unique patient identifier numbers to prevent mistakes in matching samples with patients' records
- *Productivity*: Cover the time from ordering to delivery of laboratory reports, hours of operation, phlebotomy and sample collection, laboratory layout, workflow efficiency, satellite bleeding stations for sample collection, reference laboratories, and transport methods for samples

RADIOLOGY REVIEWS

Radiology may also be called Medical Imaging if it includes not only x-rays, but also CT, MRI, fluoroscopy, ultrasound, and Nuclear Medicine. Review topics of particular concern to Radiology include:

- *Scope*: The variety of services offered and whether they are sufficient for the population and the needs of the organization, including physicians.
- *Point-of-care*: Satellite departments and portable imaging equipment that is taken to the patient's bedside facilitate access better than a central Radiology department.
- *Accuracy*: Experienced radiologists must be available to identify abnormal findings and stage tumors.
- *Productivity*: Cover the time from the order to generation of a report, and list the number of patients accommodated, hours of operation and staffing, cost-effectiveness, and patient satisfaction with services.
- *Safety measures*: Describe how staff, patients, and others are protected from excess radiation, injury, and pain.

PHARMACY REVIEWS

Pharmacy reviews must consider the broader context of medication management throughout the organization, rather than just the processes within the Pharmacy. Topics for review include:

- Use of evidence-based practices in building the formulary
- Procedures and safeguards for administration of medications, including identification of drugs through labeling, bar-coding, or other methods, and matching to appropriate patients
- Compliance with regulations and accreditation standards
- Error rates in dispersion and administration of drugs
- Education and training provided to staff about new medications/ treatments
- Procedures for ensuring medication safety and proper storage
- Policies for investigational or off-label medications
- Point-of-care in providing prescribed medications
- Efficiency and time from order to medication delivery

NURSING REVIEWS

Nursing reviews evaluate registered nurses and licensed practical nurses in relation to accreditation standards, which vary slightly from one state to another. Nurses must focus on providing good quality care. Topics for review include:

- Ethical behavior and respect for patients' rights.
- Infection control methods.
- Effective collaboration with physicians and other healthcare providers.
- Clear, legal, informative, and timely medical record documentation.
- Adherence to nursing standards, and competency.
- Data collection and measurements.
- Staff-patient ratios in different departments.
- Orientation, training, continuing education, nursing licensure and certification.
- Safety, including prevention of patient falls, injury, and ulcers, and proper administration of medications.
- Incident reports.

- Patient assessments and nursing diagnoses.
- Pain management.

GOVERNMENT REGULATION DEALING WITH COMPLAINTS, GRIEVANCES, AND APPEALS

Complaint: A specific oral or written report of lack of satisfaction with the quality of care or processes of care by a patient, guardian, or non-union staff member; a written complaint is the first step in a civil or criminal court proceeding.

Grievance: A formal written complaint about contract violation, quality of care, or financial issues by a union member.

Appeal: When a complaint or grievance is found invalid by an organization, the complainant or grievor asks for an impartial review of the decision from a third party.

Healthcare organizations that participate in federal programs, such as Medicare or Medicaid, must have procedures in place for patient complaints, grievances, and appeals as a Condition of Participation. Under this regulation, the governing board assigns a team to receive all complaints, rather than an individual. Patients must be notified of their right to file complaints, grievances, and appeals. Additional state regulations vary.

COMPLAINT ANALYSIS

A process for filing complaints, grievances, and appeals must be in place in healthcare organizations. Performing and/or coordinating **complaint analysis** includes investigation and response. These are the CPHQ's related duties:

- Receive formal complaints by the designated process, usually in writing.
- Categorize complaints by type of complaint and department or area of concern.
- Establish a timeframe for complaint resolution.
- Assign the complaint to the appropriate department.
- Investigate quality care issues, including a medical record review, interviews with those involved in the process, and onsite observations.
- Review any bylaws or regulations that may impact decisions.
- Generate reports and respond to the complaint.
- Maintain the confidentiality of files.
- Communicate with upper management, leadership, and Risk Management.
- Provide guidance for performance improvement based on findings.
- Prepare remedial training materials and present training classes.

PATIENT/CUSTOMER SATISFACTION

Patient/customer satisfaction is usually measured with *surveys* given to patients on discharge from an institution or on completion of treatment. One problem with analyzing surveys is that establishing *benchmarks* is difficult because so many different survey and data collection methods are used that comparison data may be meaningless. Internal benchmarking is more effective, but the sample rate for surveys may not be sufficient to provide validity. As patients become more knowledgeable and their demand for accountability increases, patient satisfaction is being used as a guide for performance improvement, although patient perceptions of clinical care do not always correlate with outcomes. Survey results provide feedback that makes healthcare providers more aware of customer expectations. Currently, surveys are most often used to evaluate **_service_** elements of care, rather than clinical elements. Analysis includes:

- Determining the patient/customer's degree of trust.
- Determining the degree of satisfaction with care/treatment.
- Identifying unmet needs.
- Identifying patient/customer priorities.

Reportable Events

Communication is a critical issue in incident investigation because accurate information must be collected and disseminated in a timely manner:

- Notify the investigation team members of the incident immediately, so they can begin to assist with the investigation, according to their role in the team.
- Notify all physicians, managers, administrators, and staff who are involved. Ask them to assist by reporting new incidents. Update them frequently.
- Contact the Laboratory very early in the investigation. Alert the Lab staff to save specimens as necessary for further testing. Laboratory staff can provide information about laboratory procedures that are germane to the incident.
- If necessary, notify and involve ancillary staff, such as housekeepers or food workers.
- Notify city, county, state, or federal officials, as the type of incident requires.

The CPHQ's role in **facilitating communication** with accrediting and regulatory bodies includes:

- Understanding the preferred method of communication (electronic [email, messaging], telephone, personal contact, postal mail) and to whom or what department communication should be directed.
- Utilizing the correct format for communication.
- Keeping abreast of all changes and compliance issues that may need to be addressed.
- Maintaining open communication with administration and others who deal with compliance issues and reporting any changes or issues of concern.
- Anticipating the need for more information or clarification.
- Maintaining a timeline and monitoring activities, tracking survey and reporting dates.
- Communicating at the appropriate time.
- Consulting others about issues of concern and actively seeking input.
- Greeting and orienting surveyors to the facility and introducing to key stakeholders.
- Preparing notes and talking points for administrators and others involved in compliance.

Performance, Process, and Quality Improvement Training

PERFORMANCE IMPROVEMENT TRAINING

Follow these steps for organizational **performance improvement training**:

- Perform a needs assessment and be mindful of the organizational outcomes to be achieved.
- Pretest the staff's current level of knowledge for targeted information.
- Use strategic goals to establish specific learning goals and objectives tied to the mission and vision of the organization.
- Determine methods of outcomes measurement.
- Assess staff learning styles (visual, auditory, kinesthetic) and teaching techniques to developing teaching strategies.
- Develop course materials.
- Train instructors or assistants as necessary.
- Pilot test training materials and the program with a small group and use their feedback to make modifications.
- Implement the revised training program.
- Measure to determine outcomes.

ADDIE MODEL OF ORGANIZATIONAL PERFORMANCE IMPROVEMENT TRAINING

The American Society for Training and Development developed the **ADDIE Model** for instructional systems development. It provides an outline for development of training programs in five steps:

1. ***Analysis:*** Assess the needs of the organization, the current level of knowledge, and the specific types of staff training needs, including goals and outcomes. Obtain information about needs from those involved in targeted processes. Identify the training facilities, resources, and any limitations. Develop learning objectives.
2. ***Design:*** Plan the training based on what the learners already know and need to know. Clarify the strategy for instruction and course format in a written instructional plan.
3. ***Development:*** Create course materials based on the analysis and design plan. Present the course for review to ensure it is accurate and complete. Pilot the course and review it again.
4. ***Implementation:*** Provide a training timeline and schedule of courses. Book classrooms and enroll learners. Coordinate with supervisors to ensure staff can attend classes. If extra instructors are needed, train them. Print or purchase course materials. Prepare certificates or participation records. Arrange for A/V equipment, computers, Internet access, and travel plans as necessary.
5. ***Evaluation:*** Pretest and posttest learners to find if the course material was retained. Distribute a satisfaction survey for immediate feedback about whether learners liked the course and felt it met their expectations and the stated goals. Remember that long-term outcomes related to actual performance improvement are more difficult to quantify and may take months.

FACILITY'S ORIENTATION PROGRAM

The CPHQ's participation in the **facility's orientation program** signals the administration's commitment to performance improvement. The CPHQ should not design stand-alone orientation classes, but should integrate orientation with other presentations so that the new hires understand how performance improvement is a multidisciplinary focus of the facility. Cover specific procedures, such as hand hygiene and barrier precautions, in detail. Give general information about surveillance and indicators. Staff must understand the processes in place for both patient and staff safety, and what action Human Resources will take if staff does not comply with performance improvement measures. New hires should know what all departments do to focus on process improvement, rather than just their own department.

FACILITATING AWARENESS OF DIVERSITY ISSUES AMONG STAFF

Cultural diversity is an integral part of the care plan, so always address it during in-service training. Do not assume all members of an ethnic or cultural group share the same values. Assess the patient's individual variations, and ethnic group. Make basic cultural guidelines available to staff, which outline appropriate:

- Eye contact
- Proximity
- Gestures
- Family dynamics (e.g., in patriarchal Mexican culture, the eldest male speaks for the patient. In Muslim cultures, females resist care by males.)
- Use of traditional healers or cultural medicines that must be incorporated into a care plan
- End-of-life care

Arrange for **translators** in case of language barrier, to ensure adequate communication. Get an emergency contact list of **religious visitors** (priests, rabbis, mullahs, etc.) from Chaplaincy. Ensure religious visitors are orientated, have hospital photo IDs, and parking passes. Understand and accept the attitudes and beliefs of the patient in relation to care and treatment, and treat all patients and family members with respect.

TAILORING CARE DELIVERY TO MEET THE DIVERSE NEEDS AND STRENGTHS OF PATIENTS

Diverse patients who are **ethnic, cultural or life-style minorities** often receive less than optimal care from healthcare workers. The CPHQ ensures all diverse patients and their families receive equal quality care by helping staff deliver care *tailored* to meet the individual needs of their patients. Begin by asking staff to examine their own attitudes. Hold an open discussion about diversity to help staff gain self-awareness, and determine if their ideas are stereotypical or based on spotty knowledge. Format care plans to specifically address diversity issues, so that discussions of diversity and preferences are part of care plan development, and not an addendum. The initial patient assessment should include questions about family, country of birth, educational level, religious preferences, and native language, with explanations about why the questions are asked, to establish a relationship of trust and respect. Encourage the patient and family to express their individual differences.

DEVELOPING CULTURAL DIVERSITY PLANS USING EXPERIENTIAL KNOWLEDGE

Acceptance and responsiveness to diversity requires an organizational commitment with ongoing in-service training to assist staff. The CPHQ can develop:

- *Multicultural advisory committees* with community representatives to provide insight and determine areas for research or outreach to diverse groups.
- *Mentors or consultants* who provide guidance to staff dealing with diversity issues.
- *Adaptation* of patient information, surveys, and family materials for diverse groups (e.g., culturally appropriate adaptations, translation into various languages for readers who are not proficient in English, pictorial direction signs).
- *Hiring, retention, and promotion strategies* to build a diverse workforce that is representative of the community it serves.
- *In-service training* on how to work with interpreters.

- *Integrated cultural content* throughout the training curriculum, with specific information about cultural attitudes toward intimacy, sexuality, end-of-life, mental and physical illness, drug use, and general health.
- *Presentations*, group or panel discussions that include diverse representatives.

TOTAL QUALITY MANAGEMENT (TQM)

Total Quality Management (TQM) is a quality management philosophy that promises to meet the needs of *all* customers within an organization. TQM promotes continuous improvement and quality in all aspects of an organization. TQM's goals are to increase customer satisfaction, productivity, and profits through efficiency and cost reductions. TQM requires:

- Information regarding customers' needs and opinions.
- Involvement of staff at all levels in decision-making, goal setting, and problem solving.
- Management's commitment to empower staff.
- Management's accountability through active leadership and participation.
- Teamwork with incentives and rewards for accomplishments.

The focus of TQM is on working together to *identify and solve problems,* rather than assigning blame, through an organizational culture that focuses on the needs of the customers.

14 POINTS FOR QUALITY MANAGEMENT

W. Edwards Deming developed *14 Points for Quality Management* to assist Japan with its industrial revival after World War II, and they are now widely applied to managing quality in healthcare organizations. The points are:

1. *Create constancy:* Keep focus on the purpose — improvement of products and/or services.
2. *Develop a new philosophy:* Provide effective training to ensure that things are done right the first time without delays, errors, or inefficiencies.
3. *Stop depending on mass inspections:* Eliminate the need for mass inspections by building quality into procedures, so that inspection is at the beginning of a process, instead of at the end, in order to prevent problems.
4. *Stop focusing on profits:* Assure staff that quality is more important than price.
5. *Improve constantly:* Always strive to improve every process and decrease costs through organization-wide efforts at all levels.
6. *Institute training:* Provide regular training to all levels of employees to ensure people understand their responsibilities and how to improve.
7. *Adopt effective leadership:* Increase productivity by assisting those who need help to achieve their work goals.
8. *Eliminate fear:* Communicate effectively, so employees feel secure and not fearful of punitive action.
9. *Reduce barriers:* Encourage interdisciplinary teamwork, rather than competition between areas or departments within an organization.
10. *Eliminate slogans:* Provide staff with methods to improve, rather than exhortations about the need for improvement.
11. *Eliminate numerical quotas/goals:* Focus on quality, rather than numbers, as a means to improve productivity.
12. *Remove barriers to pride of workmanship:* Encourage the efforts of staff. Eliminate annual rating or merit systems.

13. ***Provide and encourage education***: Provide ongoing educational programs for all levels of employees within an organization to foster a desire for self-improvement.
14. ***Outline management's commitment to transforming the workplace***: Actively encourage staff to constantly strive to follow the *14 Points* and do the best that they can.

CONTINUOUS QUALITY IMPROVEMENT (CQI)

Continuous Quality Improvement (CQI) is a type of **multidisciplinary management** philosophy that applies to all aspects of an organization, including Medicine, Purchasing, and Human Resources. Epidemiologic research skills are applied to analyze multiple types of events (data collection, analysis, outcomes, and action plans) because they are based on solid scientific methods. Multi-disciplinary planning brings valuable insights from various perspectives, because strategies used in one context can often be applied to another. All departments are increasingly concerned with **cost-effectiveness** as the costs of medical care continue to rise, so the quality professional is not isolated, but is part of the whole, facing similar concerns as those in other disciplines. Disciplines are often interrelated in their functions. For example, the Human Resources Department hires personnel, but other staff monitor and train them for compliance with organizational standards.

Continuous Quality Improvement (CQI) emphasizes the organization, systems and processes within a medical institution, rather than individuals. CQI recognizes internal customers (staff) and external customers (patients) and uses data to improve processes.

CORE CONCEPTS OF CQI:
- Most processes can be improved
- Quality and success are meeting or exceeding internal and external customers' needs and expectations
- Problems relate to processes
- Variations in processes lead to variations in results
- Change can be in small steps

TOOLS FOR CQI:
- Scientific method of experimentation and documentation
- Brainstorming
- Multivoting
- Charts and diagrams
- Storyboarding
- Meetings

DEVELOPING AN INTRADISCIPLINARY AND INTERDISCIPLINARY CURRICULUM

Develop an **intradisciplinary and interdisciplinary curriculum** to improve patient outcomes and quality of care with these steps:

- ***Create***: Education can include formal classes, informal discussions as part of team meetings, handouts, and computer-assisted learning (especially for night shift workers). If time is lacking to personally develop different materials for each group on-site, ask the Human Resources Department for help, or purchase customizable training materials.
- ***Coordinate***: Consider the diverse needs of different groups and plan ways to provide education to all staff members on all shifts. Adjust work schedules, offer the same presentations at different times, and broadcast and record presentations for viewing by staff that cannot attend live presentations.

- *Implement*: Schedule training to ensure the staff has adequate notice, patient care is covered, and schedules are adjusted so all can participate.
- *Evaluate*: Ask each participant to complete a course evaluation form. Evaluate the ongoing education process and make periodic evaluations of outcomes to ensure goals were met.

PROCESS IMPROVEMENT

Quality process improvement's primary principle is that advances can be accomplished in **small, incremental steps**. In large organizations with many employees, process improvement is a formal process. In small organizations or individual departments, the basic procedures are the same, but modify procedures accordingly for fewer employees. Begin continuous quality process improvement by identifying *one* process that needs improvement. For example:

- Clearly state the problem: "Poor telephone service leads to dropped calls and miscommunications between the Lab pathologist and the Operating Room surgeon regarding cancer biopsy patients."
- Contact various telephone service providers and compare features.
- Choose a better telephone service.

When the steps to improving the telephone process are completed, immediately pick another project for improvement. *Multiple* continuous improvement projects are in process at the same time.

Education

CONDUCTING AN EDUCATIONAL NEEDS ASSESSMENT

Follow these steps for an **educational needs assessment**:

- Review job descriptions to determine all staff's educational qualifications and certifications to determine what, realistically, they should be expected to know about the subject, (e.g., Infection Control).
- Review existing job orientation and training materials to determine what staff members have already been taught about performance improvement.
- Conduct meetings with staff in different departments to brainstorm areas of concern and potential training needs.
- Meet with team leaders and department heads for their input about the need for Infection Control education.
- Pretest staff with short quizzes that ask about standard performance improvement methods to determine their basic knowledge.
- Provide questionnaires to staff to obtain information about their own perceptions of what they know or need to know about performance improvement.
- Make direct observations of staff as they work.

DEVELOPING GOALS, MEASURABLE OBJECTIVES, AND LESSON PLANS FOR EDUCATION

The performance improvement team chooses an education topic, then the CPHQ develops **goals, measurable objectives** with strategies, and **lesson plans**. Focus the class on one area, e.g., proper hand washing technique. Do not make a survey course covering a broad area, like infection control in general. For example:

- Goal: To increase compliance with hand hygiene standards in ICU
- Objectives:
  o Obtain students through posters
  o 100% compliance with hand hygiene standards at 2 weeks, 1-month, and 2-month intervals after training
- Strategy:
  o Hang posters in all nursing units, staff rooms, and utility rooms by March 1
  o Develop PowerPoint presentation and obtain Intranet access for class by May 24
  o Conduct four classes at different times from May 25–31
  o Distribute hand washing kits
- 30-minute Lesson Plan:
  o Discussion: Why do we need 100% compliance? (5 min.)
  o PowerPoint: The Case for Hand Hygiene (10 min.)
  o Discussion: What did you learn? (5 min.)
  o Demonstrate correct hand washing technique (5 min.)
  o Culture samples to show bacterial reduction (5 min.)

APPLYING PRINCIPLES OF ADULT LEARNING TO EDUCATIONAL STRATEGIES

Adults come to work with a wealth of life and employment experiences. Their attitudes toward education vary considerably, but these are the **principles of adult learning** and typical characteristics of adult learners that every instructor must consider when strategizing. Adult learners are:

- Practical and goal-oriented:
  - o Provide overviews or summaries and examples.
  - o Use collaborative discussions with problem-solving exercises.
- Self-directed:
  - o Provide active involvement and ask for input.
  - o Allow different options for achieving the goal.
- Knowledgeable:
  - o Respect their life experiences and prior education.
  - o Validate their knowledge and ask for feedback.
  - o Relate new material to information with which they are already familiar.
- Relevancy-oriented:
  - o Explain how new information will apply on the job.
  - o Clearly identify objectives.
- Motivated:
  - o Provide certificates of professional advancement and/or continuing education credit when possible.

DETERMINING APPROPRIATE TEACHING APPROACHES WITH AUDIENCE SIZE AND RESOURCES

Consider **audience size** when planning presentations because:

- Student participation is more difficult in a large class because there is no time for all to speak individually. Break the class into small discussion groups or pairs for part of the class time to increase participation. Focus the discussions so that students stay on task.
- For small groups, place chairs in a circle or sit around a table to allow students to look at each other and have more active discussions than if they sit in rows.
- Online virtual classes vary considerably in size, depending on the type of presentation and whether or not scores and replies are automated or posted by the instructor. If the online group is large, set up a chat room to facilitate the exchange of ideas.

HANDOUTS

Handouts are fixtures in classes, but many end up in the wastebasket without ever being read. Follow these tips to provide useful handouts that will be read:

- Avoid PowerPoint notes that repeat everything in the presentation; just summarize the main points.
- Distributing handouts immediately prior to a discussion ensures that most of the class will be looking at the handout instead of the speaker. Place handouts in a folder or binder. Distribute them before class so people can peruse them in advance, or as students leave the class.
- Use handouts to provide guidance or worksheets for small group discussions.
- Try poster handouts (with drawings or pictures) that can be placed on bulletin boards on the nursing units.
- Use an easily readable font, like Times New Roman 12 point, not smudged copies of newspaper articles or small print text.

DETERMINING APPROPRIATE AUDIOVISUALS FOR TEACHING WITH PHYSICAL ENVIRONMENT AND RESOURCES

When considering the appropriate **audiovisuals** and handout materials for a course, keep the **physical environment** in mind because:

- Everyone in the room must be able to hear and see. For a small room, a television screen will suffice, but use a projection screen for an auditorium.
- Turn off the overhead lights and cover windows for low-resolution projectors. Flicking lights on and off during a presentation is very distracting. Use a small portable light at the podium, or use an alternate presentation format.
- PowerPoint or other presentations that include text must be of sufficient font size to be read from the back of the room.

ENSURING APPROPRIATE AND CURRENT CONTENT IN EDUCATIONAL MATERIALS

The CPHQ cannot produce all **educational materials** personally, so give careful consideration to these factors:

- **Price** for educational materials ranges from free Government Issue to thousands of dollars for proprietary software. Decide if audiovisuals are needed, an entire course, or a series of courses. Consider the budget and then look for material within those monetary constraints online. The CDC, U.S. Dept. of Labor, libraries, and universities often have text, posters, handouts, PowerPoint presentations, and videos available for free download.
- **Quality** varies considerably, so consider the goals and objectives before choosing materials. Trust sites with .gov and .org in their addresses more than blogs or sites with advertising. Only distribute the materials if they cover all needed information in a clear and engaging manner. Find at least two reputable sources that agree on the same information.
- **Currency** is an accreditation requirement. If the material will soon be outdated because of regulatory changes, ensure it can be replaced, and tell staff when to expect updates. Cite research published within the last five years.

APPROACHES TO TEACHING

There are many **approaches to teaching**, so the CPHQ must recognize the most appropriate format and plan for flexible class times, so patient care is not diminished:

- **Educational workshops** are conducted with small groups, allowing for maximum participation, and are especially good for demonstrations and practice sessions.
- **Lectures** are for academic or detailed information, but question and answer sessions and discussion are limited. An effective lecture includes audiovisual support.
- **Discussions** are best with small groups so the audience can actively participate in problem solving.
- **One-on-one instruction** is especially helpful for targeted or remedial instruction in procedures for individuals.
- **Computer/Internet modules** are good for independent learners and night shift staff.

MEASURING PERFORMANCE IMPROVEMENT TRAINING EFFECTIVENESS WITH LEARNER OUTCOMES

When the CPHQ plans an educational offering (class, online module, workshop, manuals, brochures), he or she identifies the desired **learner outcomes** from the very beginning, so learners are aware of the expectations. The subject matter of the educational material and the learner outcomes are directly related. For example, if the CPHQ teaches a class on environmental decontamination, then one learner outcome is: "By the end of this class, you will know the difference between disinfectants and antiseptics." There may be one or multiple learner outcomes. At the end of the learning experience, determine if the learner outcomes have been achieved by a survey. Ask learners if they felt they achieved the learner outcomes. Learners give valuable feedback and guidance to the CPHQ, even if they are not as familiar with the material as the CPHQ.

BEHAVIOR MODIFICATION AND COMPLIANCE RATE

Evaluate education, like all interventions, for effectiveness. Two determinants of effectiveness are measures of behavior modification and compliance rates.

- *Behavior modification* involves thorough observation and measurement, identifying behavior that needs to be changed and then planning and instituting interventions to modify that behavior. Procedures a quality professional can use include demonstrations of appropriate behavior, reinforcement, and monitoring until new behavior is adopted consistently. This is especially important to change longstanding procedures and habits of behavior.

- *Compliance rates* are determined by observation at intervals and on multiple occasions. Outcomes are another measure of compliance; that is, if education is intended to improve patient safety and decrease infection rates and that occurs, it is a good indication that there is compliance. Calculate compliance rates by determining the number of events/procedures and degree of compliance through observation or record review.

Survey Preparation Training

COORDINATING SURVEY PROCESSES

Survey processes include accreditation, licensure, and contractual requirements. The CPHQ is responsible for coordinating survey processes. The coordinator's goals are to ensure that:

- All necessary data is collected
- The proper format is used
- The most cost-efficient method is used

In some cases, electronic data sources are **incompatible**, making it impossible to transfer data, and the costs of new software can be considerable. Take a thorough inventory of all performance measures and data collected across the organization:

- Send a data inventory questionnaire to all departments, requesting information about their types of data and reasons for its collection.
- Organize the inventory results according to:
  o Core measures
  o Outcomes
  o Processes
- List definitions of the data types, storage methods, job titles of persons responsible for collections, and legal uses of the data.
- Match a complete list of all required measures against the inventory to verify compliance. It is at this point that duplications or deficiencies should become evident.

KEEPING SURVEY-READY

The **survey processes coordinator** must ensure the organization is in a constant state of survey readiness through:

- ***Identification of Leadership***: Ask the governing board to identify an administrative team and clinical leaders who will assume the responsibility for continuous readiness.
- ***Monitoring***: When the Board assigns appropriate interdisciplinary teams to monitor readiness, ensure those responsible meet four times yearly to review the organization's compliance with standards.
- ***Structure and Activities***: Document the type of administrative and team structure used for survey readiness, including team activities and responsibilities.
- ***Tracer Methodology and Performance Measures***: Conduct some form of mock survey or self-assessment *regularly*. Evaluate performance measures and intervene as necessary.
- ***Information and Communication***: Distribute standards and guidelines to leaders for reference. Flag changes in standards. Review the surveyors' reports for the last two full surveys to determine if previous recommendations have been instituted. Communicate compliance standards to staff via corporate intranet, newsletters, and in-service training sessions.

CONTINUOUS READINESS FOR ACCREDITATION

Continuous readiness means that an organization meets or exceeds the minimum accreditation and regulatory standards at all times. Facilitating survey readiness includes:

- **Coordination:** The Board appoints an administrative team with authority over continuous readiness. Identify senior leaders in each survey area, who ensure compliance. Assemble teams for quality activities to review standards and compliance.
- **Monitoring:** Interdisciplinary teams use different types of tracer methodology to evaluate a patient's progress through the system and evaluate processes. Teams meet regularly to review compliance. Conduct walkabouts regularly. Use interviews or focus groups to gather information.
- **Evaluation:** Assess all monitoring activities with software appropriate for finding patterns, trends, causes, and opportunities for improvement. Track specific performance measures and review them regularly.
- **Intervention:** Evaluate data to drive interventions. Schedule pre-surveys as early as possible in order to implement changes.

MAINTAINING KNOWLEDGE READINESS FOR ACCREDITATION

Inform: Distribute standards, explanatory material, and updates to team leaders, area leaders, and individuals involved in the accreditation or regulatory processes. Identify and apprise staff of annual changes in standards or survey processes.

Review: Review previous surveys. List previous recommendations that require action. Make action plans. Review all focused survey reports and progress reports. Review previous and current performance improvement evaluation reports to ensure recommendations are implemented.

Identify: Spotlight new compliance issues, such as annual National Patient Safety goals.

Evaluate: Determine the current status of all performance improvement activities and outcomes. Scrutinize supporting data to ensure it is adequate.

Determine: Ascertain compliance with ethics and anti-fraud policies. Scrutinize patient safety issues and the need for changes in patient safety program.

Revise: Review and revise policies and procedures as needed, to ensure consistent standards apply organization-wide.

PRE-SURVEY PREPARATION

Pre-survey preparation involves periodic self-assessment in order to evaluate compliance with standards and to prepare for *on-site surveys*:

- Organize walkabouts in all departments and areas, and focus on selected standards.
- Assemble focus teams to monitor selected standards.
- List standards on a grid, with the appropriate documentation format to show compliance
- Develop a complete electronic record or binder to outline each function or standard, with necessary references.
- Delegate tasks related to recommendations.
- Document all process improvement activities with one type of form.
- Educate those involved in process improvement.

- Inform staff of compliance issues and ensure all are familiar with the survey process and their roles.
- Review personnel records for proper credentialing, record of orientation, and completeness.
- Network with other CPHQ's about surveys.

USING TRACER METHODOLOGY FOR ACCREDITATION

Tracer methodology looks at the continuum of care a patient receives from admission to post discharge. The accreditation surveyors will use it during their visit. Test the organization's readiness by emulating the surveyors. Select a patient to trace, using his medical record as a guide.

Use the experiences of this patient, as told in documents and interviews, to evaluate the processes in place at the organization. For example, the patient selected received physiotherapy, so as a mock surveyor, begin by scrutinizing:

- *Physiotherapist*: How did the PT receive the doctor's order and arrange for patient transport? How was physiotherapy administered? How was progress noted?
- *Porter*: How did the porter receive the transport request? How long did transfer take? What route was used? What method was used to transport this patient? How was transport equipment cleaned afterwards? What do porters do if an emergency arises during transport?
- *Nurse*: How did the nurse notify the PT of the doctor's order? How did the nurse prepare the patient? How did the nurse know the therapy schedule? How did the nurse coordinate the patient's physiotherapy with other treatments? How did the nurse learn about the patient's progress?

Disseminating Improvement Information

COMMUNICATING FINDINGS

All members of an organization should be provided access to **performance improvement · information** with which they are involved. Management must ensure that confidentiality is maintained, so remove patient identifiers and practitioners' names from the data. Peer review activities must follow state regulations. Store peer review records separately from those disseminated. Provide reports to upper management and the governing board at quarterly meetings. Ask managers to disseminate reports through staff meetings. Also provide an annual summary report that tracks progress. Give teams, departments, and leaders feedback on performance measures. Use newsletters, e-mail, or the Intranet to post performance information. Include contact information for those who wish to comment or ask questions, which encourages organization-wide participation. Ask the IT Department how to ensure that sensitive information does not leave the organization by electronic means.

CHANGES IN POLICIES, PROCEDURES, AND WORKING STANDARDS

Changes in **policies, procedures, or working standards** are common, and the CPHQ is responsible for effectively educating the staff about changes related to processes in a timely manner:

- *Policies* are usually changed after a period of discussion and review by administration and staff. Make all staff aware that a policy change is under discussion. Disseminate preliminary information to staff regarding the issue during meetings or through printed notices.
- *Procedures* are connected to policy changes and are made to increase efficiency or improve patient safety, often as the result of surveillance and data about outcomes. Advertise procedural changes with posters, explain them in workshops with demonstrations, and give handouts to reinforce training.
- *Working standards* are changed in accordance with regulatory or accrediting requirements. Cover working standards extensively with discussions, workshops, and handouts so staff clearly understands the implications of non-compliance.

COMPILING AND WRITING PERFORMANCE IMPROVEMENT REPORTS

Establish formal procedures for compiling and writing **performance improvement reports** for each department or area with reporting responsibilities. Include the timeline for reports (usually monthly or quarterly). Summarize monthly reports in quarterly master reports. Written reports should include:

- Applicable organization-wide data
- Data relevant to the reporting entity
- Department-specific data for comparisons (e.g., diagnoses, demographics, morbidity, infection rates, stay lengths, external reviews, unplanned events, complaints, and incident reports)

Update and compile data at least *monthly*, even if reports are given only quarterly, so that sentinel events or outcome changes are noted and early interventions conducted. Present all reports with graphics to demonstrate comparisons. Write narratives to describe procedures. Discuss the impact of the data. Tie data to the strategic plan and goals of the organization, so that the report clearly outlines what the purpose of the data is in relation to the master plan.

TEAM REPORTS

Team reports are central to performance improvement. Written documentation must include:

- **Team charters** outline essential information about each team (operating dates, members, advisors, purpose, goals, measures, and expected outcomes). The degree of detail varies, but each charter must contain all pertinent information, such as financial and resource needs, and financial impact on the organization.
- **Quarterly and annual reports** for each performance improvement project. Begin with a statement of the desired outcomes. List process tools. Provide information about the status of the project, including data sources, and analysis methods and results.
- **Summary reports** presented in an accessible manner (electronically, in poster form, or on a storyboard). Clarify the problem with a description of actions, outcomes, and evaluation. Use charts, dashboards, or graphs whenever possible, to provide a graphic explanation.

KEY CONCEPTS OF QUALITY CARE

Quality care is:

- **Appropriate** to needs and follows best practice standards.
- **Accessible** to everyone, despite financial, cultural, or other barriers.
- **Competent,** with well-trained practitioners who adhere to standards.
- **Coordinated** among all healthcare providers.
- **Effective** in achieving outcomes, based on the current state of medical knowledge.
- **Efficient** in its methods for achieving the desired outcomes.
- **Preventive,** allowing for early detection and prevention of problems.
- **Respectful**, so that the individual patient's needs are given primary importance.
- **Safe,** so that the organization is free of hazards or dangers that put patients, visitors, and staff at risk.
- **Timely**, ensuring the correct care is provided on time.

Communicate these **key concepts** to all members of the organization through in-service training, workshops, newsletters, fact sheets, and team meetings.

USING INTERNAL RESOURCES AND THE EXPERTISE OF OTHERS

Assisting staff to understand and **use internal resources and the expertise of others** requires a commitment of time and effort:

- Coach others on methods of collaboration. Provide handouts about effective communication strategies. Model collaboration with the staff being coached.
- Conduct team meetings for departments, where collaboration is modeled, and suggest the need for outside expertise to help with patient care planning. Initiate discussions about resources that are available within the facility (e.g., medical library; university affiliates; in-house trainers; bilingual staff; expert users) and the community (e.g., Public Health; Emergency Medical Services; Red Cross; immigrant settlement services; women's groups; disease-specific support groups).
- Select diverse teams that reflect the catchment area, or invite **subject matter experts** (SME, pronounced *"smee"*) to mentor teams when needed.

Communication

ACTIVE LISTENING AS PART OF THERAPEUTIC COMMUNICATION

- **Therapeutic communication** begins with respect for the patient and his or her family.
- **Make a personal introduction**, use the patient's name, and listen intently.
- **Use open-ended questions** like: "Is there anything you'd like to discuss?"
- **Acknowledge comments** by nodding or stating, "Yes, I understand."
- Reflect statements back; e.g.,
  - Patient: "I hate it here!"
  - Staff: "You hate it here?"
- Use reflection sparingly.
- Make observations, like:
  - "You are shaking."
  - "You seem worried."
- Recognize the patient's feelings:
  - Patient: "I want to go home."
  - Staff: "It must be hard to be away from your family and friends."
- **Allow silence** and observe non-verbal behavior, rather than force conversation.
- **Provide information** as honestly and completely as possible about the patient's condition, treatment, and procedures.

THERAPEUTIC COMMUNICATION PHRASES PROMOTING CARING AND SUPPORTIVE ENVIRONMENTS

Here are some **therapeutic communication phrases** that support patient care:

- Express implied messages:
  - Patient: "This treatment is too much trouble."
  - Staff: "You think the treatment isn't helping you?"
- **Explore a topic**, but allow the patient to terminate the discussion without further probing: "I'd like to hear how you feel about that."
- Indicate reality:
  - Patient: "Someone is screaming."
  - Staff: "That sound was an ambulance siren."
- **Comment on distortions** without directly agreeing or disagreeing:
  - Patient: "That nurse promised I wouldn't have any shot!"
  - Staff: "Really? That's surprising because this medicine can only be given as an injection."
- **Work together**: "Maybe if we talk about this, we can figure out a way to make the treatment easier for you."
- Seek validation:
  - "Do you feel better now?"
  - "Did the medication help you breathe better?"

AVOIDING NON-THERAPEUTIC COMMUNICATION

While using therapeutic communication is important, it is equally important to **avoid interjecting non-therapeutic communication**, which blocks effective communication. *Avoid the following:*

- Meaningless clichés:
  - "Don't worry. Everything will be fine."
  - "Isn't it a nice day?"
- **Providing unsought advice:** "You should..." or "The best thing to do is...." Patients accept advice better if they *ask* for it. Provide facts and encourage the patient to reach a decision.
- **Inappropriate approval** that prevents the patient from expressing true feelings or concerns:
  - Patient: "I shouldn't cry when Mommy goes home."
  - Staff: "That's right! You're a big boy!"
- **Asking for explanations** of behavior that is not directly related to patient care and requires analysis and explanation of feelings: "Why are you crying?"
- **Agreeing with, rather than accepting and responding** to patient's statements, makes it difficult for the patient to change his or her statement or opinion later: "I agree with you," or "You're right."

Seven examples of **non-therapeutic communication** are:

- **Negative judgments:** "You should stop arguing with the nurses."
- **Devaluing patient's feelings:** "Everyone gets upset at times."
- **Disagreeing directly:** "That can't be true," or "I think you are wrong."
- **Defending against criticism:** "The doctor is not being rude, he's just very busy today."
- **Subject change** to avoid dealing with uncomfortable topics:
  - Patient: "I'm never going to get well."
  - Staff: "Your parents will be here in just a few minutes."
- **Inappropriate literal responses**, even as a joke, especially if the patient is at all confused or having difficulty expressing ideas:
  - Patient: "There are bugs crawling under my skin."
  - Staff: "I'll get some bug spray."
- **Challenge to establish reality**, which often just increases confusion and frustration: "If you were dying, you wouldn't be able to yell and kick!"

INTERNAL COMMUNICATION DUTIES

The quality professional fulfills organization-wide **communication duties** by:

Reviewing communications related to process improvement, reports, and feedback to determine if:

- The governing body and staff are familiar with strategic goals and successful improvement processes.
- Each staff member is aware of his or her personal responsibilities for patient safety.

Providing communications organization-wide, in an easily accessible format, such as:

- Ensuring policies and procedure manuals are on-line.
- Making calendars with timelines for reports and other process improvement activities.
- Sending e-mail reminders.
- Giving regular reports and updates at department, management, and team meetings.
- Communications are in a variety of formats, such as newsletters, e-mails, screensavers, and FAQ sheets.

EMPOWERING STAFF AND PATIENTS

One goal of patient management is to **empower staff** with the tools they need to establish an environment of mutual respect. Empowering others does not mean that management loses authority or the leadership role. Rather, management shares responsibilities and works with staff to set goals and establish a clear vision for the organization. Empowerment includes encouraging participation in policy-making and allowing staff members to take active roles in patient management. Empowerment requires an investment in time and education, so staff is properly trained to assume responsibility, and have a clear understanding of the parameters of their authority. Staff members must feel that they have the support of management. **Empower patients** and their families by allowing them to participate in decisions about their care and to receive respect.

PROBLEM SOLVING

Problem solving in any medical context involves arriving at a hypothesis and then testing and assessing data to determine if the hypothesis holds true. When a problem arises, these steps help avoid a recurrence:

1. *Resolve* the immediate problem.
2. *Define* the larger issue by talking with the patient, his or her family, and staff to determine if the problem related to a failure of communication or other issues, such as culture or religion.
3. *Collect data* by interviewing additional staff or reviewing documents, to gain a variety of perspectives.
4. *Identify important concepts* to determine if there are issues related to values or beliefs.
5. *Consider reasons for actions* to distinguish the motives and intentions of all parties, which underlie the problem.
6. *Decide* how to prevent a recurrence of the problem, based on patient advocacy and moral agency; reach the best solution possible for the patient and family.

Ethics

RESOLVING ETHICAL AND CLINICAL CONFLICTS

Ethical and clinical conflicts among patients and their families and healthcare professionals are not uncommon. Issues frequently relate to medications and treatment, religion, concepts of truth-telling, lack of respect for the patient's autonomy, limitations of managed care, or incompetent care. Healthcare providers are in a position to easily manipulate patients and their families by providing incomplete information and influencing decisions. The CPHQ questions and listens, acknowledges each person's perspective, and shares different viewpoints. ***Open communication*** is critical to resolving conflicts. Ask what steps could be taken to resolve the conflict or how it could be handled differently. This often leads to compromise because it allows for an exchange of ideas and validates legitimate concerns. Sharing cultural perspectives can lead to better understanding. Advocacy for the patient and family must remain at the center of the CPHQ's conflict resolution technique.

PROMOTING AN ENVIRONMENT CONDUCIVE TO ETHICAL DECISION-MAKING AND PATIENT ADVOCACY

An **environment** suitable for ethical decision-making and patient advocacy does not appear spontaneously during a crisis; it requires planning and preparation. The institution must clearly communicate that nurses are legally and morally responsible for assuring competent care and respecting the rights of patients. Decisions regarding ethical issues often must be made quickly, with no time for contemplation; therefore, immediately discuss ethical issues as they arise. The CPHQ must:

- Ensure the policies and procedures manual clearly defines how to deal with conflicts.
- Assemble an active Ethics Committee.
- Provide in-service training.
- Discuss ethics at staff meetings.

Patients and families need to be part of the ethical environment, and that means empowering them by providing information (print, video, audio) that outlines patient's rights, the procedures for expressing their wishes, and dealing with ethical conflicts. Respect for privacy and confidentiality, and a non-punitive atmosphere are essential.

INCORPORATING PATIENT AND FAMILY RIGHTS INTO ACTION PLANS

Patient and family rights must be incorporated into action plans. Design the action plan collaboratively and encourage participation from patients and family members. Include patients and families on advisory committees. Use assessment tools, such as patient and family surveys, to gain insight into the issues that are important to them. Infants and small children cannot speak for themselves, so the CPHQ must act as their advocate. Include not only the immediate family, but also other groups or communities who have an interest in patient care (e.g., local AIDS committee). Many hospital stays are now short-term, so programs must include follow-up interviews and assessments to determine if the needs of the patient and family were addressed in the care plan.

ROLE MODELING, TEACHING, COACHING, AND MENTORING

These different approaches help develop nurses' **advocacy,** moral agency, and caring practices:

- ***Role modeling*** takes place when one nurse serves as an ideal example for others, demonstrating the behavior and responses that advocate for the patient and show caring practices. The nurse observes, interviews, attempts to understand the patient/family's perspective, and intervenes to assure that their needs are met.

- **Coaching** is providing staff with tools, responses, or procedures that help them to advocate.
- **Mentoring** is providing professional guidance to a staff member who has questions or concerns, and acting as a resource.

EMPOWERING PATIENTS AND FAMILIES TO ACT AS THEIR OWN ADVOCATES

Empower patients and families to act as their own advocates by giving them a clear understanding of their rights and responsibilities in print or an audio/video presentation on admission, or as soon as possible thereafter:

- **Rights** include competent, non-discriminatory medical care, respect for privacy, participation in decisions about care, and the right to refuse care. Give clear, understandable explanations of treatments, options, and conditions, including outcomes. Explain transfers, changes in care plans, and advance directives. Give access to medical records, and information about charges.
- **Responsibilities** include providing honest, thorough information about health issues and medical history. Encourage them to ask for clarification if they don't understand the information provided to them and to follow the plan of care that is outlined, or explain why that is not possible. They should treat staff and other patients with respect.

INTEGRATING CONCERNS AND VALUE SYSTEMS INTO A PATIENT'S PLAN OF CARE

The CPHQ must understand what is **most important** to the patient, family, staff, administrators, and payers in the plan of care. Participants have widely divergent concerns. Integrating their various perspectives is an ongoing effort, as it is impractical to call a participant meeting to discuss each care plan. Identify general concerns and values for the institution or the unit, and individualize them for each patient. For example, the:

- Child wants her parents be with her at all times.
- Parent wants religious and cultural concerns about medical care to be respected.
- Insurance company wants appropriate, cost-effective treatments.
- Nurse wants treatments clearly outlined and carried out competently.
- Nutritionist wants the child to have appropriate TPN.
- Radiologist wants to minimize the child's exposure to x-rays when placing nasogastric tubes.

An adequate care plan allows all of these concerns to be addressed.

ETHICS AND PAIN MANAGEMENT

Promoting a caring and supportive environment means ensuring that the patient is comfortable. According to Joint Commission guidelines and federal law, all patients have the right to **pain management**, and this applies to infants and children too.

- Assess pain management procedures already in place to determine their effectiveness or need for change.
- Establish the minimum standard that should be legally followed.
- Ensure a pharmacist, anesthetist, and nurses collaborate on an updated pain management policy and procedure.
- Clarify responsibility for pain control and imbed this in the standards of practice, e.g., involve oncologists, surgeons, rheumatologists, and other specialists who prescribe analgesics and anesthetics.
- Train staff about guardrails to reduce pain safely.

- Educate patients to understand they are entitled to pain control, rapid response, and the benefits of pain management.
- Promote the new pain management policy and procedure organization-wide.

Health Data Analytics

Maintaining Confidentiality

CONFIDENTIALITY

Maintaining **confidentiality** of performance improvement activities, records, and reports is mandated by state and Federal **regulations**:

- The **Health Insurance Portability and Accountability Act (HIPAA)** protects patients' right to privacy and confidentiality of patient records. An organization can use patients' records for internal quality performance activities, such as monitoring for infections, without obtaining a specific, written authorization signed by the patient or guardian. The governing board, healthcare personnel involved in direct patient care, supervisory staff, and quality teams are allowed access to patients' medical information. When patient information is part of records or reports that will be shared externally, remove the identifying patient information.
- The **Healthcare Quality Improvement Act (HCQIA)** provides privacy protection for healthcare organizations and personnel engaged in formal peer review procedures, such as accreditation and performance improvement activities, because confidentiality and immunity further the quality of healthcare. Exclude identifying information from reports and records. Certain conditions apply, and personnel are not exempted from lawsuits for criminal actions.

REQUIRED CONFIDENTIALITY AGREEMENTS AND CONFLICT OF INTEREST STATEMENTS

The CPHQ must inform staff about regulations and correct reporting methods to maintain the confidentiality o**f performance improvement activities and records**. When staff members understand confidentiality issues, it lessens some of their concerns about their performance reviews. Most organizations require personnel who review medical records or participate in performance improvement activities to sign *confidentiality agreements,* which outline privacy issues and increase awareness of confidentiality concerns. Each healthcare organization must have a *conflict of interest policy* in place to ensure that reviewers are not primary care givers, and do not have an economic or personal interest in a case under review. Limit access to protected health information to those who need the information to complete their duties related to direct care, or to performance improvement review activities.

MAINTAINING THE CONFIDENTIALITY OF PERFORMANCE-RELATED DATA

Performance improvement teams generate **reports** on a regular basis, which can be monthly, quarterly, or annually, depending on the size of the institution, the population numbers, or device days. Statistics must include adequate *denominator data* for meaningful analysis, and this can require a longer period of time. Specific data about individual patients and healthcare workers are protected by privacy laws (e.g., HIPAA), so do not disseminate information about individuals unless their anonymity is assured. Provide *confidential reports* to individual physicians about their own effectiveness rates. When presenting comparison rates, do not identify the other physicians. Present reports to the administration, teams, and staff in the areas surveyed. Thus, if a quality study involved an ICU, make the ICU staff and physicians aware of the study results, so they can evaluate the effectiveness of their procedures or institute preventive methods.

Data Collection Plans

PERFORMING/COORDINATING DATA INVENTORY LISTING ACTIVITIES

To perform or coordinate **data inventory listing** for information management:

- Assemble a team that includes members knowledgeable about data management and assign them to the inventory.
- Develop a procedure and a reporting grid that includes the type of data, its source, reasons for collection, the receiver, storage method, and its uses.
- Inventory from the top down, because the organization has multiple sources of data
- Catalog data in this order:
  o **Accreditation** (e.g., core measures)
  o **Licensure** (e.g., infection rates and staffing ratios)
  o **Contracts** (e.g., utilization costs)

DEPARTMENTAL

INDIVIDUAL UNITS

- Include everything that is counted, even if it simply involves a clerk counting the use of Foley catheters to facilitate ordering supplies because this data relates to other measures, such as urinary infection rates.
- Once the inventory is completed, assess the grid for duplications, deficits, and unused data.

PERFORMING/COORDINATING OF DATA DEFINITION ACTIVITIES

Data definition activities are a necessary step in performance improvement. Data definition must be completed as part of the planning process and included in the written plan, using input from quality teams or other sources. Every aspect of data collection requires definition. For example, when measuring infection rates, define what constitutes an infection. Save time by incorporating definitions from the CDC, industry, or accreditation standards. For example, use the Joint Commission's definition of infection, with subtypes of iatrogenic, endemic, epidemic, and health-care associated infections.

Outcomes are changes in health status, for example:

- A decrease in mortality
- Changes in behavior or knowledge, such as a diet modification used to control diabetes
- Positive surveys indicating satisfaction with treatment

Outcome definitions are especially important, because outcomes allow progress to be assessed. With any measurement, the outcome must indicate what expected change will occur in response to performance improvement activities.

DATA COLLECTION METHODOLOGY

Correct **data collection methodology** is comprehensive and encompasses all aspects of performance improvement activities. As the data collection coordinator, the CPHQ ensures that the:

- Data collection staff is selected based on their knowledge and access.
- Collection begins with a complete inventory of existing data.
- Data collection is systematic.
- Unnecessary data collection and duplication of effort is avoided.

- Interdisciplinary teams who are knowledgeable about the performance improvement process identify sources of data and guide collection.
- Triggers are set.
- Most effective data collection method is used.
- Data is integrated to help identify patterns or trends (organization-wide and departmental).
- Definitions and collection methods used are based on sound principles of epidemiology ensuring the right type of data is collected.
- Frequency and duration of data collection is determined based on actual needs.

POPULATION AND SAMPLING

A **population** is a particular group of individuals, objects, or events. Gather data on either an entire population or a subset of a population within a specified time frame. For example, if all cases of a particular disease, all deaths, or all physicians in a particular discipline are measured, it involves an entire population. **Sampling** measures only a subset of a given population and generalizes the findings to the larger target population. Consider these factors when sampling:

- The sample must have the characteristics of the target population.
- The design of the collection must specify the size of the sample, the location, and time period.
- The sampling technique must ensure that the sampling represents the target population accurately.
- The design of the collection must ensure that the sampling is not biased.

Defining the population is critical to data collection and the criteria must be established early in the process.

PROBABILITY SAMPLING

Probability sampling occurs when there is an equal chance for any member of a group to be part of the sample, allowing generalization of results to the entire population. Probability sampling is usually more expensive than non-probability. There are six sub-types of probability sampling.

- **Cluster:** The target population is divided into clusters or groups, and then a number of these groups are selected at random and all members of the population within the selected groups are sampled.
- **Multi-stage:** This method is similar to cluster. However, all members of the population in selected groups are not sampled. Instead, a sampling of the selected groups is used. Use any method for choosing members of a population, such as simple random sampling.
- **Simple random:** The cases in a given population are chosen randomly, using a standard Table of Random Digits. This is the easiest and most commonly used method of sampling.
- **Stratified:** Two-tier sampling. Divide a group into strata (mutually exclusive groups) with two or more homogenous characteristics. Sample a specified number from each stratum. Thus, outpatient surgery patients with intravenous solutions are sampled by diagnosis, solution, length of stay, or complications.
- **Systematic (interval) random:** Select the first member of the population randomly; select other members at regular intervals. E.g., the desired sampling is 100:500, so the *sampling interval* is 5 (1 in 5). Choose a random number between 1 and 5 as the *random start*. Sample every fifth member to a total of 100 (20 members).
- **Multi-phase:** Two phases are required, but more can be used. Obtain data from an entire specified population. Based on that data, obtain further data from a subgroup within the original population.

CONFIDENCE LEVEL AND NON-PROBABILITY SAMPLING

Depending on the goal of data collection, different **types of sampling** or combinations of sampling may be utilized. Sampling should have a **confidence level** of 95% (.05 level), meaning that there is a 95% chance that the sample represents the population and results can be replicated. Types include non-probability and probability.

- **Non-probability** sampling is intentionally biased (not everyone has an equal chance of being included) and results cannot be generalized to an entire population. It utilizes qualitative judgment.
- **Convenience sampling** is a type of opportunity sampling when those available are sampled, such as all patients in an STD clinic on a Tuesday.
- **Quota sampling** utilizes a stratified population that is divided into subgroups (such as male and female) and then a proportion is sampled, such as 5% of females over 16 with HIV. Sometimes specified numbers are counted, such as 50 males and 50 females.
- **Purpose sampling** utilizes members of a particular population, such as all women over 60 with breast implants.

ISSUES WITH DATA DEFINITION AND COLLECTION OF DATA

Data definitions must be based on a solid understanding of statistical analysis and epidemiological concepts. Specific issues that must be addressed include:

- 3 S's:
  - **Sensitivity:** The data must include all positive cases; Accounting for variables decreases the number of false negatives.
  - **Specificity:** The data must include only those cases specific to the needs of the measurement, and exclude those that are similar but different population, decreasing the number of false positives.
  - **Stratification:** Data is classified according to subsets, taking variables into consideration.
- 2 R's:
  - **Recordability:** The tool or indicator must collect and measure the necessary data.
  - **Reliability:** Results should be reproducible.
- UV:
  - **Usability:** The tool or indicator should be easy to use and understand.
  - **Validity:** Collection must measure the target adequately, so that the results have predictive value.

Selecting Software

USING COMPUTERIZED SYSTEMS TO ANALYZE DATA

The analysis of data by hand is impractical and time-consuming, unless the surveyed population is very small. Most statistical analysis utilizes **computer software programs** to automatically analyze the data in a number of different ways and account for risk factors. Software programs save time by generating numeric data, text reports, and graphs simultaneously. The amount and type of data that must be entered into a program varies, according to the type of software and the necessary data for reports that will be generated. If different programs are used to collect and analyze data, they must be *compatible*, so that data moves intact from one program to another to generate reports. *Data-entry design* is important: *Fields* in which numeric data is entered are calculable; fixed numbers (telephone, birth date, medical record numbers, and Social Security) are entered as text.

SELECTING SOFTWARE FOR DATA COLLECTION

Software selection and evaluation of hardware requires knowledge, time, and financial commitment on the part of the organization. The requirements are:

- **Commitment:** Administration and staff must agree to the financial outlay and to the learning curve as part of the strategic plan.
- **Team selection:** Choose an interdisciplinary team with members who are knowledgeable about data, hardware, and software to evaluate the proposed programs. Educate this team about the performance improvement process. Have them conduct a data inventory first, to determine needs organization-wide and avoid duplication.
- **Identification of system requirements for the organization:** Review the whole organization to determine the current extent of its technology (number, types, and locations of computers) and the ability of the technology to interface. Assess organization-wide goals and needs, barriers to implementing an integrated system, and future needs.
- **Identification of user needs**: Gain staff participation through questionnaires, checklists, surveys, group meetings, brainstorming, and wish lists. Relate needs to the strategic plan. Prioritize them to identify essential needs.
- **Assessment of current systems:** Contact the IT Department. Find out if:
  - Staff use current hardware well.
  - Proposed software can interface with current software.
  - Downloads are safe and secure data exchange is possible.
  - Data storage is protected to comply with HIPAA.
  - Current computer capacity is adequate.
  - Proposed software is easy to access, input data, and produce reports.
- **Evaluation of vendors:** Internet search, network, and attend conferences about the kind of software needed. Send a *Request for Proposal* to vendors to facilitate comparison. Get references from vendors as evidence that they effectively implemented the proposed program with similar organizations. Vendors must provide a product history that includes: Frequency of upgrades; compatibility with previous software versions; advice about product maintenance and service upgrades.

- **Evaluate and compare different software programs**: Perform a software evaluation in relation to the identified needs of the organization. Decide which specifications must be met. Write a Request for Proposal (RFP) to outline the needs of the organization. Although many vendors will not provide a customized response to an RPF unless the budget is large, the team can use it as a guide and checklist during the evaluation process. When comparing software, ask:
  o Does this program meet our organization's requirements?
  o Is it appropriate for medical needs?
  o Is it compatible with our existing hardware?
  o Is it cost-effective, based on our cost/benefit analysis?
  o Can we visit similar organizations that already use this software, to see it in action?
- **Negotiate a contract:** Always review several vendor contracts prior to completing one. Each contract must include provisions for delivery, installation, training, support, liabilities, prices, payment terms, program modifications, and confidentiality. *Seek legal advice.*

EVALUATING COMPUTER HARDWARE AND SOFTWARE INTENDED FOR DATA COLLECTION AND ANALYSIS

Performance improvement teams must survey, analyze and take action quickly if outbreaks or clusters of infection occur. Drawbacks that slow their emergency response time include:

- Manual record keeping and reporting
- Lack of integration among existing computer **hardware and software programs** (e.g., Laboratories use one program, but nursing units use another that is incompatible.)
- High cost of integrating all computer systems and software

Hire a consultant with expertise in **medical hardware and software** to advise about the best solution to keep data safe, per HIPAA regulations. Before hiring a software designer to create a custom program to meet specific needs, ensure that it can communicate with existing reporting and other software. If the organization buys generic programs and equipment, budget for expensive upgrades every two years, including the time it takes IT to install and teach users about the upgrades. If selecting Web-based programs because patches and upgrades download automatically, ensure the workstations are Internet capable, and budget for antivirus software.

Always review hardware along with software, to ensure the needs and their uses are compatible. **Centralized hardware systems** include:

- Mainframes (a large central computer system with terminals)
- Shared systems (leased computers outside the facility)
- Networks with a server and client computers

Decentralized hardware systems are:

- Unattached to a central computer
- Connected by local area networks (LANS) or wide area networks (WANS)
- Linked through the telephone or Internet

Evaluate hardware for:

- Cost
- Operating system types

- Type and amount of memory storage (internal, CD, digital video discs, shared off-site, Web storage, optical disks, external hard drives)
- Flexibility
- Capability
- Current needs

IMPLEMENTING NEW COMPUTER SYSTEMS

Implementing a new computer system for data collection and analysis requires considerable training and a transitional period:

- **Prepare:** Announce the new system organization-wide before installation. Explain how the system benefits the entire organization and relates to the strategic plan. Provide information to staff tailored to fit each area's needs. Give a timeline for transition to the new system.
- **Train:** The type and need for training varies, depending on the individual's responsibility in relation to the computerized system. Make training hands-on, in small groups, and repeat classes at various times, so staff achieves mastery, rather than familiarity. Provide area managers with additional training (expert user level) to assist in them in supervising.
- **Supervise:** Once the system is in place, supervise staff to ensure that it is used correctly. Identify problems in use to modify the training curriculum. Stay alert for problems (e.g., staff visiting porn sites, selling patient information to the media, applying for external jobs during work time, or cyber stalking).

COSTLINESS OF INCOMPATIBLE DATA ENTRY SYSTEMS

If different **computerized data entry systems** are not integrated, it increases costs for data collectors and Medical Records. For example, if lab reports and nursing notes use incompatible systems, then data collectors duplicate efforts by transcribing them, and Medical Records must print all patients' charts. Hard copy storage wastes space and requires more clerks. Three ways to enter data are:

1. **Manual data entry**, the most common method, which means charting directly into the computer or copy typing written information. Make responsibilities for entering data clear, to prevent backlogs. Thoroughly train staff in correct procedures for data entry. Expect errors due to transpositions and entering data on the wrong chart.
2. **Scanners**, programmed to read particular forms, such as those with boxes marked in pencil. Optical character recognition (OCR) software scans hard copies into computerized text, so that external reports can be added to the system without retyping.
3. **PDA's**, which transfer data collected in the field to a desktop computer, rather than re-entering data from forms by hand.

Epidemiological Theory and Surveillance

USING EPIDEMIOLOGICAL THEORY IN DATA COLLECTION AND ANALYSIS

Epidemiology studies the relationship between the frequency and distribution of diseases to determine causes, especially of infectious outbreaks and poisonings. The Society for Healthcare Epidemiology of America (SHEA) is an industry leader in promoting the use of epidemiology for healthcare to reduce infections and improve quality of care. Epidemiology focuses on ***populations*** or ***cohorts*** of patients, rather than on individuals, so it is especially valuable in relation to data collection and analysis. Use epidemiological data to:

- Assess and compare different clinical practices.
- Determine good system design.
- Develop criteria for measurement, including outcomes and comparative analysis of data.
- Design quality control measures.
- Document response to changes.

DETERMINING THE PREVALENCE OF EPIDEMIOLOGICALLY SIGNIFICANT FINDINGS

While **incidence** counts *new* events, such as infection diagnosed during a given time period, **prevalence** (proportion) counts *existing* infections, regardless of when the disease was contracted, during a specified period of time (period prevalence) or at a point in time (point prevalence). Prevalence is a good measure of the overall burden of infections/events on a facility, expressing how common they are. Prevalence is often expressed as a percentage.

In ***limited-duration prevalence***, prevalence is looked at *retrospectively*. It counts all those alive during a period of time (e.g., the past 5 years) who had a particular disease.

Complete/lifetime prevalence, on the other hand, counts all those alive at a *particular point* in time who had the disease at any time in the past or present, whether cured or in current treatment, usually expressed as a ratio of those with the disease, compared to a given population.

GENERATION, ANALYSIS AND VALIDATION OF EPIDEMIOLOGICAL SURVEILLANCE DATA

Most **generation of data** is from available resources, such as admissions records, questionnaires, interviews, medical records, public health reports, and laboratory reports. In some cases, data generation is part of the surveillance process. For example, urine cultures may be done routinely as part of a surveillance plan, or threshold rates may generate further testing. Perform ***analysis*** in a timely manner, because it is especially important for the detection of outbreaks. The type of analysis depends on the expected outcomes and the purpose of surveillance. ***Validation*** of data is an ongoing process. Review all steps in the generation and analysis of data regularly, especially when threshold rates are exceeded. If, for example, an apparent outbreak of antibiotic-resistant bacteria is detected in wound cultures, then validate the nurses' swab collection procedure *and* the laboratory technologists' culture plating procedure, to ensure that the outbreak is not a pseudo-epidemic caused by faulty techniques or deviations in Infection Control.

USING RISK STRATIFICATION IN EPIDEMIOLOGICAL SURVEILLANCE STUDIES

Risk stratification involves statistical adjustment to account for confounding issues and differences in risk factors. ***Confounding issues*** are those that confuse the data outcomes, such as trying to compare different populations, different ages, or different genders. For example, if there are two physicians and one has primarily high-risk patients and the other has primarily low-risk patients, the same rate of infection (by raw data) would suggest that the infection risks are equal for both physicians' patients. However, high-risk patients are much more prone to infection, so in this case, risk stratification to account for this difference would show that the patients of the physician with low-risk patients had a much higher risk of infection, relatively speaking. Risk stratification is also used to predict outcomes of surgery by accounting for various risk factors (including ASO score, age, and medical conditions). Risk stratification is an important element of data analysis.

TARGETED SURVEILLANCE

Targeted surveillance is limited in scope, focusing on particular types of infections, areas in the facility, or patient populations. It is less expensive than hospital-wide surveillance and may provide more meaningful data, but clusters of infection outside the survey parameters are missed. Targeted areas are picked based on characteristics such as frequency of infection, mortality rates, financial costs, and the ability to use data to prevent infections:

- *Site-directed* targets find particular sites of infection, such as the bloodstream, wounds, or urine
- *Unit-directed* targets select particular service areas of the hospital, such as intensive care units or neonatal units
- *Population-directed* targets scrutinize high-risk groups, such as organ transplant patients
- *Limited periodic* targets combine hospital-wide surveillance of all infections for one month in each quarter, followed by site-directed targets for the rest of the quarter. This increases the chance of detecting clusters of infection, but those that fall outside of the hospital-wide surveillance months are still missed.

Selecting Measures

DEVELOPING OBJECTIVE PERFORMANCE MEASURES

The development of **objective performance measures** is critical to monitoring performance improvement. Most organizations have many types of data, but often it is not in a usable form for performance improvement. Identify **data needs** first. Categories of performance measures include those needed for:

- *Strategic planning* (specific to the organization).
- *Regulations* (to meet state or federal requirements).
- *Contractual agreements* (as in managed care).

Consider all three of these categories when developing performance measures, to avoid duplication, and to ensure that the data collected will evaluate the effectiveness of the organization. The data provided should directly relate to **functions** and **processes**. Basically, two types of measurements are required:

- *Outcomes*, which show how the organization is performing and whether or not goals are being achieved. For example, data may measure mortality rates in a Neonatal Intensive Care Unit.
- *Processes*, which show if the organizational systems/functions are working effectively. For example, data may measure compliance with core measures for accreditation.

SELECTING PERFORMANCE MEASURES

Below are **areas of concern when selecting performance measures**:

- *Responsibility for selection*: Each team should select appropriate performance measures. There may be a number of different teams selecting measures for different levels, such as organization-wide data, as opposed to departmental data. These teams are usually interdisciplinary and members have training or expertise in utilizing performance measures.
- *Clear understanding*: Functions, processes, and variables that may affect outcomes require standardized language, a glossary, and consistent training
- *Identification of purpose and utilization*: Data may be used to assess quality, or for accountability, or for research
- *Review and inventory*: There must be current, available data within the organization's databases to determine what can be utilized
- *Measures*: Determine the numerators, denominators, and measures that will be used. Assess the measures for their reliability and validity and document these findings. Post the definitions, and list reasons for their choice and references for each measure.

SELECTING OUTCOME MEASURES

Process and **outcomes** are equally important in performance improvement. Consider whether to focus on the process or the outcome. Establish both a short-term and a long-term focus for outcomes.

- *Short-term outcomes* show results directly related to the process, allowing for modifications of the process.
- *Long-term outcomes* relate more to general quality of care and patient satisfaction, and are used retrospectively to evaluate the process or plan for future care.

91

Outcomes do not directly assess process, although they serve as an indicator that a process may be effective or ineffective, requiring further study or modification of process. Planners focus on identifying three types of outcome measures:

- **Clinical**: Determines if there are positive results from clinical interventions
- **Customer functioning**: Includes indicators of ability to *perform*
- **Customer satisfaction**: Includes meeting expectations and needs

Developing Scorecards

BALANCED SCORECARD

The **balanced scorecard** (designed by Kaplan and Norton) is based on the strategic plan, and provides performance measures in relation to the mission and vision statements, and goals and objectives. A balanced scorecard includes not only the traditional financial information, but also includes data about customers, internal processes, and education/learning. Each organization can select measures that help to determine if the organization is on track in meeting its goals. These measures may include:

- *Customers*: Types of customers and customer satisfaction.
- *Finances/business operations*: Financial data may include funding and cost-benefit analysis.
- *Clinical outcomes*: Complications, infection rates, inpatient and outpatient data, compliance with regulatory standards.
- *Education/learning*: In-service training, continuing education, assessment of learning and utilization of new skills, research.
- *Community*: Ongoing needs.
- *Growth*: Innovative programs.

If the scorecard is adequately balanced, it will reflect both the needs and priorities of the **organization** itself, and also those of the **community and customers** it serves.

DASHBOARD

A digital **dashboard**, like the dashboard in a car, provides an overview of an organization. A dashboard is an easy to access and read computer program that integrates a variety of performance measures or key indicators into one display, usually with graphs or charts. It might include data regarding patient satisfaction, infection rates, financial status, or any other measurement that is important to assess *performance*. The dashboard provides a running picture of the *status* of the department or organization at any point in time, and may be updated as desired—daily, weekly, or monthly. An organization-wide dashboard provides numerous benefits:

- Broad involvement of all departments.
- A consistent and easy to understand visual representation of data.
- Identification of negative findings or trends so that they can be corrected.
- Availability of detailed reports.
- Effective measurements that demonstrate the degree of efficiency.
- Assistance with making informed decisions.

Collecting and Validating Data

TRIGGERS

Triggers are mechanisms or signals within data that indicate when further analysis or prioritizing must be done, such as case reviews or root-cause analysis. Select triggers for each measure of performance.

Data Triggers:

- **Sentinel events:** Unexpected death or major impairment lasting at least two weeks, occurring because of a process or system deficiency.
- **Adverse events (AE):** An unintended, unfavorable, iatrogenic occurrence that is life-threatening, or requires in-patient hospitalization, or extends the patient's length of stay, or causes a birth defect or lasting disability.
- **Performance rate:** Pre-established level of performance in a particular measure.
- **Rate change:** A pre-established change over a specified time period.
- **Difference between groups:** A pattern of disparity between specified groups.
- **Specified upper and lower control limits about a mean:** Guardrails establish an acceptable range of variation, usually set by standard deviation methods.

External Triggers:

- Feedback from staff, internal and external customers
- Strategic planning initiatives; practice guidelines
- Benchmarks; research

IDENTIFYING EXTERNAL AND INTERNAL DATA SOURCES

As part of the data inventory process, all sources of data must be identified, including **external and internal data sources**.

Internal sources are those that originate within the organization. These are numerous and some are easy to overlook, so review all departments for data. Internal sources include: Patients' records; patient and staff surveys; medications records; clinical review reports (medication use, mortality rates, and autopsy reports); admissions data (demographics); laboratory reports; observation reports; Infection Control reports; team and case management reports; financial statements; environmental safety reports; minutes of meetings; and utilization review reports.

External sources originate outside the organization and may reflect activity within or outside the organization. External sources include: Reference databases; accreditation reports; CDC reports; state reviews; scientific and medical literature reviews; state or nationally-identified best practice reports; threshold data; comparative data; sentinel event alerts; third-party (payer) reports; and national guidelines.

INTERNAL AND EXTERNAL VALIDITY

Many surveillance plans are most concerned with **internal validity** (adequate, unbiased data properly collected and analyzed within the population studied). However, studies that determine the efficacy of procedures or treatments should also have **external validity** (the results should be generalized and true for similar populations). Replicating the study with different subjects, researchers, and under different circumstances should produce similar results. For example, some people are excluded from a study, so that instead of randomized subjects, the subjects are highly

94

selected. When data is compared with another population in which there is less or more selection, results are different. The selection of subjects, in this case, interferes with external validity. Part of the design of a study should include considerations of whether or not it should have external validity, or whether there is value for the institution based solely on internal validity.

QUALITATIVE AND QUANTITATIVE DATA

Both qualitative and quantitative data are used for analysis, but their focus is quite different:

- **Qualitative data:** Data are described verbally or graphically, and the results are subjective, depending on observers to provide information. Interviews may be used as a tool to gather information, and the researcher's interpretation of data is important. Gathering qualitative data is time-intensive, and it usually cannot be generalized to a larger population. Qualitative information gathering is useful at the *beginning* of the design process for data collection.
- **Quantitative data:** Data are described in terms of numbers within a statistical format. Quantitative information gathering occurs *after* the design of data collection is outlined, usually in later stages. Tools may include surveys, questionnaires, or other methods of obtaining numerical data. The researcher's role is objective.

DATA NEEDED FOR ANALYSIS TO ASSIST WITH STRATEGIC PLANNING

Four types of data must be analyzed and summarized to assist with strategic planning:

- *Medical/clinical* information is patient-specific and includes patient history, diagnosis, treatment, laboratory findings, consultations, care plans, physician orders, signed informed consents, and advance directives. The medical record should include records of all procedures, a discharge summary, and emergency care records.
- *Knowledge-based* information is:
  o Methods that ensure staff is trained and supported
  o Research
  o Library services and access to information
  o Good practice guidelines
- *Comparison* data makes internal or external comparisons to benchmarks or best-practice guidelines.
- *Aggregate* data includes pharmacy transactions, required reports, demographic information, financial information, hazard and safety practices, and most things not included in the clinical record.

Data Measurement and Analysis

ORGANIZATIONAL TRANSPARENCY

Organizational transparency is a fairly new concept for the healthcare industry, which has been better known for concealment of data. Public pressure to make healthcare organizations more transparent arose in response to unnecessary surgery, inflationary costs, high infection rates, and other negative information in the press. The organization must commit to transparency of *pricing* and *quality*, so that both staff and patients have realistic expectations of care. Information that should be available in the reports includes:

- Financial **costs** and **profits.**
- **Performance measures**: Clearly outline the factors that are valued and measured.
- **Outcomes**: List both positive improvements and negative failures to improve to demonstrate quality control is in place.
- **Safety records**: Summarize safety concerns for dissemination, but do not identify those involved without their written permission.
- **Medical records** are open to individual patients and guardians.
- **Leadership qualities** that are parameters for promotion.

RELATION OF FEDERAL EXECUTIVE ORDERS TO ORGANIZATIONAL TRANSPARENCY

In August 2007, President Bush signed the *Executive Order to Help Increase the Transparency of American's Health Care System*. It applies to all federal and federally-sponsored health programs, and stresses that patients have a right to know about quality and pricing when purchasing healthcare. It provides a series of goals to:

- Increase transparency in *pricing*, including the costs of procedures.
- Increase transparency in *quality*, including information on the quality of services provided by doctors, hospitals, and other healthcare providers.
- Encourage adoption of *health information technology (IT) standards* to increase and improve rapid exchange of health information.
- Provide options that promote *quality* and *efficiency* in healthcare.

At present, no measures are mandated. However, the federal government recognizes that healthcare organizations must become more transparent if they are to compete effectively and provide the type of care patients need and expect.

WEB SITE CONTENT FOR ENSURING ACCURACY IN PUBLIC REPORTING

When designing a Web site, consider:

- Who is your audience?
- What type of machine will most viewers use to access your site?
- What type of information do they want?
- Are your code and server secured?
- Are copyright and privacy issues addressed?
- Is access open, or are sections restricted through passwords?
- Who will be the contact for viewer feedback in each section?
- Who updates information for each area or department?
- Is the site primarily informational, educational, or both?
- What format and navigation system are best for your audience?

- How much and what type of direct marketing is included?
- Do interactivity and hi-res graphics slow down page loading?
- Are your typeface and language readable by a large audience?
- What technology is supported (e.g., PDF, Flash, cookies, hit counters, forms, encryption, on-line credit card payments)?
- Is the site well-designed and easy to use?

External Reporting

PATIENT SAFETY INDICATORS

The Agency for Healthcare Research and Quality (AHRQ) has developed **Patient Safety Indicators** (sets of specific quality indicators), regarding the potential for complications and adverse events for patients receiving treatment. AHRQ has sponsored the development of surveys for assessment of patient safety for different healthcare organizations, including hospitals, nursing home and outpatient facilities, and provides free software to allow the organization to compute its AHRQ quality improvement rate. Patient safety indicators include:

- *Provider-level indicators:* Include such indicators as pressure ulcer rate, retained surgical items, CLABSI, postoperative hip fracture, postoperative sepsis, and transfusion reaction count.
- *Area-level indicators:* Include such indicators as retained surgical item, iatrogenic pneumothorax rate, and postoperative hemorrhage/hematoma rate.

Hospitals may participate in data collection for research. For example, those participating in data collection regarding rates of CLABSI, submitted data for entry into the AHRQ database each month directly or through the CDCs National Healthcare Safety Network (NYSN).

HEDIS BUNDLED PAYMENTS

HEDIS bundled payments are based on the healthcare provider's HEDIS score, so accurate reporting is essential. With bundled payments (also called **episode payments** or **episode-based payments**), payments are received by healthcare providers in a lump sum in advance of care for specific conditions or courses of treatment. This allows healthcare providers to focus on the patient's plan of care rather than reimbursement. The better the patient outcomes, the better the healthcare profit because every complication adds to cost of care. Bundled payments may cover multiple services and service providers. Each organization must report specific HEDIS measures and results of the HEDIS/CAPHS (Consumer Assessment of Healthcare Providers and Systems) survey each year. The organization's measures and survey results are compared to national benchmarks and regional and national thresholds. Data for the preceding year is reported in June, so data from January 2017 to December 2017 would be reported in June 2018, utilizing the appropriate ICD-10 and CPT coding.

Data Management Systems and Data Display

ORGANIZING THE AGENDA, REPORTS, AND MINUTES FOR COMMITTEE MEETINGS

Organize the agenda, reports and minutes in a meeting to involve and inform the **committee** members:

- *Agenda*: Distribute the agenda electronically to all interested parties 2–3 days prior to a meeting. Itemize the agenda and include the names of people giving or receiving reports. List approximate times for discussion beside each item, especially if there are many agenda items. If the agenda is for a report to upper management or the governing board, summarize the results of performance improvement activities with a dashboard.
- *Reports*: Schedule reports early in the meeting to allow for discussion, as they may relate to other agenda items. Prepare an electronic presentation with PowerPoint® or an overhead projector to summarize complex issues.
- *Minutes*: Distribute minutes within 2–3 days after the meeting. Minutes must include brief summaries of each agenda item.

If the organization does not already have standard formats, save time by downloading easy to use agendas, reports, PowerPoint® presentations, and minutes templates free from Microsoft at: http://office.microsoft.com/en-us/templates/.

AGGREGATION AND SUMMARY OF DATA

Data must be **aggregated** and **summarized** for correct analysis of results. Identify those responsible individuals or groups, and the time frame for processing and reporting the data. As the data is collected, display the data on a dashboard or in another manner that demonstrates the type of problems, their extent, and causes. Write a report that summarizes findings and reaches conclusions based on the data. Display data in a graph to make it accessible. Performance improvement professionals must generate reports on a regular basis. Choose monthly, quarterly, or annually, depending on the size of the institution and the population numbers or device days. Statistics must include adequate denominator data for meaningful analysis, which can delay report generation.

CHARTS AND GRAPHS

Presenting data in the form of **charts and graphs** provides a visual representation of the data that is easy to comprehend. There are basically 3 types of graphs: line, bar, and pie.

- *Line graphs* have an *x*- and *y*-axis, so they are used to show how an independent variable affects a dependent variable. Line graphs show a time series, with time usually on the *x* (horizontal) axis. Use line graphs to show the number of infections per week/month.
- *Bar graphs* compare and show the relationship between two or more groups. The graphs show quantifiable data as bars that extend horizontally, vertically, or stacked. Bar graphs compare data from different populations or from one time period to another.
- *Pie charts* show what percentage an item pertains to the whole. Use a pie chart to show distribution of infection control resources.

Common chart and graph software programs are Microsoft Excel, Corel Quattro Pro, and Quicken. If examples of dashboards are required for executive summaries, visit: https://www.idashboards.com/.

PARETO CHARTS

A **Pareto chart** is a combination vertical bar graph and line graph. Typically, bar graph values are arranged in descending order. For example, if incidences of bloodstream infections are plotted by unit, then the unit with the largest number appears first on the left. A line graph superimposed over the bar graph shows what accumulated percentage of the total is represented by the elements of the bar graph. Thus, if 50 infections occurred in the ICU, and that represented 30% of the hospital's total infections, the line graph starts at 30%. If 40 infections occurred in the Transplant Unit, the line graph shows 24%. Pareto charts demonstrate the most common causes or sources of problems, and have given rise to the 80/20 rule: 80% of the problem often derives from 20% of causes.

FLOW CHARTS

A **flow chart** is a quality improvement tool used to provide a pictorial or schematic representation of a **process**. When searching for solutions to a problem, analyze each step in a process and post it on the flow chart. *Use the following standard symbols:*

- Parallelogram: Input and output (start/end)
- Arrow: Direction of flow
- Diamond-shape: Conditional decision (Yes/No or True/False)
- Circles: Connector joining two parts of a program; divergent paths with multiple arrows enter, but only arrow exits

Flow goes from top to bottom and left to right. Flow charts help audiences visualize how a process is carried out and examine a process for problems. Flow charts are used to plan a process before its inception. Flow charts demonstrate critical pathways to outline treatment options and paths related to findings. Examples of flow chart programs are Microsoft Visio, Corel Flow, and ABC Flowcharter. If these programs are not accessible, obtain free trial software at http://www.smartdraw.com/ or http://www.gliffy.com.

ISHIKAWA FISHBONE DIAGRAM

The **Ishikawa fishbone diagram** resembles the head and bones of a fish. It is an analysis tool that determines **cause and effect** and is used for brainstorming. In performance improvement, it identifies root causes. Label the "head" with the problem (effect). Label each "bone" with one of these categories (causes):

- **M** for manufacturing, methods, materials, manpower, machines, measurement, and Mother Nature (environment)
- **P** for people, prices, promotion, places, policies, procedures, products, and administration
- **S** for service, surroundings, suppliers, systems, and skills

The categories serve only as a guide and are selected and modified as needed.

RUN CHARTS

The **run chart** is a type of line graph with a horizontal x-axis (independent variables) and vertical y-axis (dependent variables, outcomes). The run chart provides a running record of a process over time when a horizontal median line is added, calculated according to the number of data points (data points + 1 divided by 2). A *run* is a sequence of data points on one side of the median line, ending when the line crosses the median. Runs should be color coded. For example, a run chart may plot the number of urinary infections by month for a one-year period with increased runs indicated by a different color. Record data for a long enough period, so that normal variations are not misconstrued as significant runs.

Run charts with more than 25 data points demonstrate:

- **Shifts** (≥8 points on one side of the median line)
- **Trends** (6 data points in the same direction)
- **Patterns** (≥8 similar fluctuations)

If any of these three changes appear, they point to specific causes that require investigation.

CONTROL CHARTS

The **control chart** is similar to the run chart but has a mean line (the average of the data points) as well as upper and lower control limit lines, based on normal distribution. Every process has some normal variation (***common cause or random variation***), so the line values may vary, but when the line crosses the control limits, this suggests that there is a specific cause (***special cause variation***) that requires investigation. The control limits are usually set at 2–3 standard deviations from the median. Thus, the line shows the normal variations and excessive variations. The control chart can include horizontal lines indicating each standard deviation for more precise information, dividing the graph into zones. Zone C is 1 standard deviation from mean, Zone B is 2 standard deviations from mean, and Zone A is 3. Positive values are above the mean line and negative values are below it. Analyze the data for specific trends, depending on the number of data points in each zone.

SCATTERGRAM

A **scattergram** graphically displays the correlation between two variables, with one variable represented on the x-axis and the other on the y-axis.

- Each plotted data point indicates the value of both variables for a given person, event, or time period.
- If the data points show a clear tendency to go up or down when moving left to right across the graph, this indicates correlation (positive or negative).
- **Remember that correlation does not equal causation.** Just because two quantities seem to show a pattern, it does not mean that there is a causal relationship between the two. The correlation could be random, or both quantities could be influenced by some unconsidered third quantity.

REGRESSION ANALYSIS

Regression analysis compares the relationship between two variables to determine the nature of their correlation, if it exists. There are a few common types of regression analysis that can be performed, but linear regression is the most common. Regression analysis is essentially the process of comparing a set of real-world data to a mathematical model and assessing how well the data set matches the model.

The strength of a correlation relationship is indicated by the correlation coefficient (r), which ranges from +1 to -1:

- **An r-value of -1** indicates a perfect ***negative*** correlation: value of one variable decreases when value of the other increases
- **An r-value of +1** indicates a perfect ***positive*** correlation: values of both variables increase or decrease together
- **An r-value close to 0** indicates no correlation: the values of the variables change independently of one another

Statistics for Data Description

P VALUES

Surveillance is sometimes confused by randomness. A sudden increase in the infection rate at a facility does not necessarily indicate a systemic problem at the facility, but may simply be a random statistical variation. One useful metric for determining whether an observed effect is the result of random variation rather than a systemic problem is the **p value**. The p value indicates the likelihood that an observed effect is random, with values ranging from 0 to 1.

- A p value **less than 0.05** means that there is less than a 5% probability that the observed effect occurred by chance, while a p value **greater than 0.05** means that there is more than a 5% probability that the observed effect occurred by chance.
- The value **0.05** is generally considered to be the cutoff for **statistical significance**. As a practical matter, policy decisions are typically not made based on studies where the results are not found to be statistically significant.

It's important to realize though that the *p value* is just one measurement of the validity of a set of data and should be combined with other statistical analyses. A limited outbreak at a small facility may not generate enough data points to attain a statistically significant *p value*, but it can still be epidemiologically important.

INCIDENCE VS. PREVALENCE

Incidence and prevalence surveillance are both hospital-wide surveillance methods. **Incidence surveillance** is ongoing surveillance of infections of all hospitalized patients, recording the number of new infections in a population of patients over a specific period of time. Incidence surveillance is time-consuming and expensive but identifies clusters of infections and allows for risk-factor analysis.

To calculate the incidence rate:

$$\frac{\text{Number of new infections}}{\text{Total population in time period}}$$

Prevalence surveillance involves both *period prevalence*, which is a specific, pre-determined time period for surveillance, and *point prevalence*, a specific point in time. Prevalence is the number of nosocomial infection cases active during the period or point of time covered by the survey.

To calculate the prevalence rate:

$$\frac{\text{Number with active infections}}{\text{Total population in time period}}$$

RATES AND RATIOS FOR COMPILING SURVEILLANCE DATA

A **rate** is the number of events per a given population (e.g., 3 infections per 100 patients) or per a time period (e.g., 3 infections per 1,000 device days). These figures are expressed as the **ratios** 3:100 and 3:1,000. Rates and ratios express most Infection Control data. However, data should be stratified, taking risk factors into account, and different rates derived for different populations for validity. **Risk ratio** is the ratio of incidence of infection/disease among those who have been exposed, compared to the incidence among those who have not been exposed. A risk ratio of 1.0 suggests that there is equal risk of infection. A higher number suggests the probability that those exposed will have higher rates. Thus, 1.5 shows that the exposed group is 1.5 times more likely to become infected than those not exposed. A lower number suggests exposure brings less risk of infection (immunity).

CALCULATING PROPORTIONS

A **proportion** is a subset of ratio that identifies a part of the whole. The event being studied as the numerator data must be a part of the population or database used for the denominator data, for example:

$$\frac{5 \text{ urinary infections}}{40 \text{ patients with Foley catheters}}$$

Proportions are expressed as either decimals or percentages:

- Calculated as a *decimal proportion*, the above example is 5 ÷ 40 = 0.125
- Calculated as a *percentage proportion*, the above example is 5 ÷ 40 × 100 = 12.5%

Proportion is referred to as a rate when looking at data over a specified period of time. Proportion is frequently used to provide general epidemiological information about specific populations, for example, the number of smokers of different ages in a given population, such as African-American teenage boys.

MEASURES OF AVERAGES

Measures of averages locate the **center point** of a group of data:

- *Mean* is the average number. However, since distribution can vary widely, the mean may not give an accurate picture. For example, if compiling data and one unit has 20 infections per 100 and the other has 1 infection per 100 (and both have the same total number of patients), the mean (21 ÷ 2) is 10.5 per 100, which has little validity.
- *Median* is the 50th percentile. For example, consider the following numbers: 1, 3, **7**, 9, and 15. The number 7 is the median (middle) number. If there is an even number of data points, then average the two middle numbers, e.g., 1, 3, **7**, **9**, 14, and 15. The numbers 7 and 9 are averaged, so the median is 8. If there is an even distribution, the mean and median will be the same. The wider the difference between the two, the more uneven the distribution.
- *Mode* is the number occurring with the highest frequency. There may be bi-modal or tri-modal numbers.

MEASURES OF DISTRIBUTION

Measures of distribution show the **spread** or dispersion of data:

- *Range* is the distance from the highest to the lowest number. The term *interquartile* denotes the range between the 25th percentile and the 75th percentile. Report range with median to provide information about both the center point and the dispersion.
- *Variance* measures the distribution spread around an average value. Use variance to calculate the effect of variables. A large variance suggests a wide distribution. A small variance indicates that the random variables are close to the mean.
- *Standard deviation* is the square root of the variance and shows the dispersion of data above and below the mean in equally measured distances. In a normal distribution, 68% of the data is within one deviation (measured distance) of the mean, 95% within 2 deviations and 99.7% within 3 deviations.

RATE COMPARISONS

Comparisons of rates are used to measure or analyze performance. For example, reports of nosocomial (hospital-acquired) infections are often used to compare one facility with another facility or one department in the same facility with another, such as the ICU with the Transplant Unit. *Interpret in-house comparisons carefully, because a higher rate of infection does not always mean patients are at increased risk.* To make comparisons meaningful, ensure that data is collected in the same way in different units, and case findings and supporting laboratory tests are consistent and accurate. Risk factors should be similar or results stratified to account for differences in risk factors

STATISTICAL SIGNIFICANCE OF CAUSAL INFERENCE (HILL'S CRITERIA)

In epidemiology, a statistical association is not necessarily definitive. Sir A. Bradford Hill (1897-1991) made important contributions to epidemiological research methods by developing criteria to judge a **causal inference**. The more of the following criteria that are met, the more likely that an association is *causal* (the exposure caused a disease):

- **Strength of association** as measured by a *p* value less than 0.05.
- **Temporality:** Cause must precede event.
- **Consistency of observations:** The same effect occurs in different populations and settings.
- **Plausibility of theory:** The theory is based on sound biological principles.
- **Coherence:** The theory does not conflict with other knowledge/theories.
- **Specificity:** One primary cause for an outcome strengthens causality.
- **Dose relationship:** An increase in exposure should increase the risk.
- **Experimental evidence:** Related experimental research may increase the causal inference.
- **Analogical extension:** That which is true in one situation applies to another

SPOTTING TRENDS ON A CHART

Look at the run chart or control chart to see if the data points consistently go upward or downward, indicating a clear trend. If there are many variations, then the trend is more difficult to analyze. Apply these rules of **trending analysis** to help determine if the variations are ***common cause variations*** or ***special cause variations***:

- ***Run (shift):*** 7 or more consecutive data points all above or all below the median (run chart) or mean (control chart).
- ***Trend:*** 7 or more consecutive data points in either ascending or descending order with 21 or more total data points, or 6 or more if fewer than 21 total data points were plotted.
- ***Cycle:*** Up and down variation, forming a sawtooth pattern with 14 successive data points, suggestive of systemic effect on data. If the trend is related to common cause variation, the variation is demonstrated with 4–11 successive data points.
- ***Astronomical value:*** A data point unrelated to other points indicates a sentinel event or special cause variation.

EXTERNAL BENCHMARKING AND INTERNAL TRENDING

External benchmarking involves analyzing data from outside an institution, such as monitoring national rates of nosocomial (hospital-acquired) infection and comparing them to internal rates. To make this data meaningful, use the same definitions and the same populations for effective risk stratification. Using national data is informative, but each institution is different, so relying on external benchmarking to select indicators for Infection Control or other processes can be misleading. Benchmarking is a compilation of data that may vary considerably if analyzed individually, and its anonymity makes comparisons difficult. **Internal trending** involves comparing internal rates of one area or population with another, such as infection rates in ICU and General Surgery. Trending can help to pinpoint areas of concern within an institution, but making comparisons is still problematical because of inherent differences. Use a combination of external and internal data to identify and select reliable indicators.

Interpreting Data to Support Decision-Making

INTERPRETING PERFORMANCE PRODUCTIVITY REPORTS

Performance productivity reports provide a wealth of information about the processes within an organization, but interpreting the data requires a thorough understanding of the organization and existing processes. The data may be useful for a variety of purposes:

- **To evaluate clinical processes:** Changes often require cooperation of medical staff, including physician compliance with best practices and core measures, and providing supporting data can be a powerful motivator.
- **To coordinate needs and services across the organization:** Data may, in some cases, be generalized to apply to multiple processes.

TO ASSURE AN ACCEPTABLE BALANCE OF COST-EFFECTIVENESS AND GOOD PRACTICES

- **To promote a culture of accountability:** Data provides objective information about cause/effect and outcomes.
- **To improve the flow of information:** Data can be used effectively to communicate needs and promote interchange of ideas.

PROCESS VARIATION

When interpreting performance productivity reports, the CPHQ must have a clear understanding of **process variation** to determine whether variations found in the data are within an acceptable range or are cause for concern. Some random variations are normal in-patient care processes and patient responses. For example, patients respond differently to the same treatment. Commonly caused problems are difficult to resolve and require changes in general processes, but variations can be reduced to a stable level. Assignable causes are identifiable, such as sentinel events, which are traced through root cause analysis. Deal with assignable causes individually, with case-specific reviews to identify and eliminate the cause of the variation. Variations can be positive, and then further study is needed to determine how best to replicate the beneficial practice.

OPPORTUNITIES FOR DECISION-MAKING

Opportunities for decision-making may be evident on analysis of **indicators** (typical cause events, such as infections related to central venous lines) and **outcomes** (rates of infection). Surveillance activities produce both numerator and denominator data. Measure the outcomes against established internal benchmarks or external benchmarks, such as national rates. When it is clear where variances lie, target these particular indicators for improvement. Additionally, observations or other findings may indicate the need for changes in processes. For example, cost-benefit analysis may show that some procedures or processes are not cost-effective, and there are a number of different, cheaper solutions that might achieve the same or better results. Review these alternate solutions, so that the costly processes or procedures become a target for reduction in variable costs to the facility.

CATEGORICAL DATA

Interpreting performance productivity reports requires a thorough understanding of statistical processes and measures to make reasoned judgments for using the data. Accurately interpreting data is equally important to collecting it. There are two basic types of data, categorical and continuous.

Categorical (or discrete) data is qualitative and divided into different categories, such as numbers of clinical patients, genders, events, births, and deaths. Categorical data is usually displayed in tables or bar graphs, with the total for each variable referred to as a marginal distribution. Categorical data may be presented as raw numerical data and in ordinal scales (for ranking) or used as numerators and denominator, but the statistics are easier to interpret if they are converted to percentages. Categorical data cannot be fractionated; that is, the data is presented as only whole numbers because, for example, someone cannot be half born. Categorical data can include qualitative information with nominal descriptions rather than numerical data, such as blood types.

CONTINUOUS DATA

Continuous (variable) data is quantitative data measured in both whole and fractional units, such as blood pressure readings, temperatures, and infection rates, and is often used for physical measurements. If data is expressed in fractions or decimals, then it is continuous, not categorical. Categorical data is expressed in whole numbers. Use continuous data to obtain averages (means and medians) and establish ranges and standard deviations for control charts. Continuous data is often used to establish internal benchmarks to compare with external benchmarks, such as national data, to determine how an organization differs, to identify opportunities for process improvement, and to develop effective practice guidelines.

OUTCOME DATA

When interpreting **outcome data**, keep in mind that there are a number of different types, and some data may overlap:

- **Clinical:** Includes symptoms, diagnoses, staging of disease and indicators of patient health
- **Physiological:** Includes measures of physical abnormalities, loss of function, and activities of daily living
- **Psychosocial:** Includes feelings, perceptions, beliefs, functional impairment, and role performance
- **Integrative:** Includes measures of mortality, longevity, and cost-effectiveness
- **Perception:** Includes customer perceptions, evaluations, and satisfaction
- **Organization-wide clinical:** Includes readmissions, adverse reactions, and deaths

When considering outcome data, focus on the purpose of reviewing the data, rather than on a process or the outcome data itself. The team must analyze the data to understand how process and outcome data interrelate.

INITIAL VS. INTENSIVE ANALYSES

An **initial analysis** must be conducted for every monitored process. This means identifying team members responsible for the aggregation and analysis of data, specifying timelines for aggregation and analysis of data based on the volumes of customers, services, procedures, and the impact on those involved. Once the timeline is established, the analysis should begin. Data is reviewed for accuracy and reliability and compared both internally and externally to look for trends or patterns. Data is reviewed for evidence of sentinel or individual events for further study. Triggers are set for patient safety or other areas of concern. Trigger events spark an *intensive analysis*, which is used to identify opportunities for improvement, and to identify significant deficiencies and the scope of problems.

Intensive analysis focuses on:

- Sentinel events
- Performance levels outside of normal variations
- Performance levels outside of benchmarks or best practices

107

- Hazardous conditions
- Medical discrepancies and errors

RELATION OF SELECTION BIAS AND INFORMATION BIAS TO STATISTICAL SIGNIFICANCE

Selection bias occurs when the method of selecting subjects results in cohorts who are not representative of the target population because of an inherent error in design. For example, if all patients who develop urinary infections with urinary catheters are evaluated per urine culture & sensitivities for microbial resistance, but only those patients with clinically-evident infections are included, a number of patients with sub-clinical infections are missed, skewing the results. Selection bias is only a concern when participants in studies are specifically chosen. Many surveillance studies do not involve subject selection.

Information bias occurs when there are errors in classification, so an estimate of association is incorrect.

- ***Non-differential misclassification*** occurs when there is similar misclassification of disease or exposure among both those who are diseased/exposed and those who are not.
- ***Differential misclassification*** occurs when there is a differing misclassification of disease or exposure among both those who are diseased/exposed and those who are not.

ORGANIZATION OF REPORTING AND STATISTICAL SIGNIFICANCE

The organization of reporting can result in inaccurate data if:

- ***Insufficient information*** results from incomplete medical records or lab reports at the time of survey. There may be a failure in the reporting procedure, so that some data is not reported.
- ***Evaluation errors*** occur when data is available but is overlooked, or its significance is not understood, so that the data is not included in a survey.
- ***Insufficient laboratory testing*** occurs because the attending physician receives a report that indicates clinically evident infection, but does not follow up to verify it, and threshold rates have not been established to automatically trigger a follow-up.
- ***Negligence*** makes staff reluctant to verify and report infections and negative events in order to keep their rates artificially low.

Because of differences in the efficiency of collecting data, the facility with the lowest infection rate may be the one with the least accurate collection of data.

IDENTIFYING VARIANCES THAT REQUIRE ACTION

First, ensure that **baseline data** is representative of the target population. This requires an initial period of surveillance and review, ideally for one month. Establish threshold rates. Once the baseline is established, analyze new data to identify ***variances*** (changes, like an infection increase that indicates an epidemic or a mortality decrease that indicates improvement). Predetermine a trigger for an alert. For example, if infection rates increase 2 standard deviations above the monthly mean, this variance triggers an alert. Alerts may be tied to time, so that an increase over a 3-month period triggers an alert. Once data triggers a variance alert, a statistical analysis must be completed as soon as possible to determine the:

- Relevance of the variance.
- Probability of the variance occurring by chance.
- Statistical significance or insignificance of the variance.

CHI-SQUARE TEST

The **chi-square** (X^2) is a method of comparing **rates** or **ratios**. The chi-square test establishes if a variance in **categorical** data (as opposed to numerical data) is of statistical significance. An example of categorical data is that concerning gender (male vs. female). There are a number of different approaches to chi-square testing, depending upon the type of data, but it is generally used to show if there is a significant difference between groups or conditions being analyzed. For example, use chi-square to compare the rates of surgical infections between two types of surgical procedures.

T-TEST

The **t-test** analyzes data to determine if there is a statistically significant difference in the **means** of both groups. The t-test looks at two sets of things that are similar. For example, the t-test could compare the average number of miles walked per week by women over 65 who have been diagnosed with breast cancer, as opposed to women over 65 who have not been diagnosed.

IS–IS NOT METHOD

Is–Is Not is a quality control method to identify root causes and keep the team focused on the immediate problem.

- Create a table with a header above two columns. Write the problem at the top, in the header. Title one column **"Is,"** and the other **"Is Not."**
- Ask who, what, where, when, why, and how in relation to the *process*. Do not focus on the people involved. Create a detailed description of the problem or event. When the problem or event actually IS identified, write it in the *"Is"* column.
- Ask what things could have caused the same problem, but did not. Evaluate similar processes in which the problem did not occur. When what the problem or event IS NOT is identified, write a detailed description in the *"Is Not"* column.
- Compare the two columns of information. Determine what distinguishes them to help find potential causes.
- Identify changes that occurred, resulting in the problem, which leads to a root cause.

FIVE WHYS

The **Five Whys** is a method of finding root causes and solving problems designed by Taiichi Ohno of Toyota, in Japan. This process requires a pre-trained, knowledgeable team, who asks "why" in a sequential manner, to narrow the focus and arrive at consensus about the cause of an event. The steps are:

- Outline the process in detail and describe each event in the sequence of events
- Ask "why" questions about each step in the sequence of events to try to determine cause. For example:
  - **Q:** Why did the patient return to the Emergency Department?
  - **A:** Because the doctor initially failed to order an x-ray of the patient's injured hand.
  - **Q:** Why did the doctor fail to order an x-ray of the patient's injured hand?
  - **A:** Because the Radiology Department was understaffed and there was a two-hour delay to obtain x-rays.
- Reach a consensus and propose solutions to improve performance.

INTERPRETATION OF INCIDENT REPORTS

Incident reports, also called occurrence reports, provide valuable evidence of a problem with process performance. About 50% of incident reports relate directly to **medical error**. Use incident reports to investigate the incident, provide a guide to change, provide data about occurrences, and provide legal defense related to liability claims. There are four primary types of events related to medical error:

- Near error
- Unsafe activity
- Sentinel
- Adverse

The organization must have a systematic method in place for **interpreting** incident reports, which involves not only collecting data relating to the reports, but also analyzing the data and utilizing it for educational purposes and performance improvement activities. An important function of interpretation is to determine if the incident could have been prevented, and, if so, what part of the current process failed and what can be done to prevent similar incidents in the future.

INTERPRETATION OF OUTCOME DATA

Outcome data guides performance improvement activities because it gives evidence of how well a process succeeds, but not necessarily the reasons; therefore, the CPHQ must **evaluate** the outcome data to find reasons. Consider these two inherent problems with outcome data when using outcomes for process improvement:

- It is almost impossible to provide sufficient risk stratification to provide complete validity to outcome data
- It is also difficult to accurately attribute the outcome data to any one step in a process without further study

For example: Outcome data shows a decline in deaths in the Emergency Department, which recently changed its trauma procedures. The outcome data does not take into account the local police station's gang task force, which successfully decreased drive-by shootings and killings by 70% in the catchment area. The CPHQ might assume that changes in the Emergency Department's trauma procedures altered the outcome data when, in fact, if the data were adjusted for these external factors, the death rate may have increased.

ISSUES

Tie process improvement activities and **outcome data** to each other and assess processes for their cost-effectiveness. For example: An initial cost-benefit analysis determined an intervention was necessary in Infection Control. The governing board agreed to implement a proposed intervention by investing $93,000 per year, expecting a savings of 5 infections at $135,000 ($43,000 net). After one year, the CPHQ carefully assess the outcomes to determine if the intervention met the goal set for it and it was cost-effective. They discover that the savings only amounted to only 2 infections at $34,000 each. Then, the added cost to the hospital is $59,000. However, do not base *changes in practice* solely on monetary figures. Perform further analysis to determine if other variables affected the outcomes. If the hospital opened a transplant unit with additional surgical patients, then the reduction in 2 infections might be impressive. If there is a *Staphylococcus* carrier among the staff, then this might account for additional infections. In some cases, a change of practice is required.

MODELS OF INTEGRATION

Integrating the results of data analysis into the performance improvement process varies from one type or size of organization to another, depending on the **model of integration** that the organization uses:

- *Organizational*: Processes for improvement are identified and teams are selected to participate in different areas or departments. Teams report to the same individual, who monitors progress.
- *Functional/coordinated*: Staff specialties, such as Risk Management and Quality Management, are not integrated. They remain separate, but draw from the same data resources to determine issues related to quality of care and efficiency.
- *Functional/integrated*: Staff specialties remain, but there is cross-training among specialties, and a case management approach to patient care is used, so that one person follows the progress of a patient through the system and coordinates with the various specialties, such as Infection Control and Quality Management.

INTEGRATING PERFORMANCE PRODUCTIVITY REPORTS INTO THE PERFORMANCE IMPROVEMENT PROCESS

Performance productivity reports are a beginning point in efforts to improve performance. The reports must be analyzed to determine what areas of improvement have the most impact on strategic goals and outcomes related to goals. Prioritize needs. Use the reports as a basis for improved performance in these ways:

- **Education and training**: Inform staff about the results of the reports, because making people aware of how well they are doing and what areas need improvement provides an impetus for change. Develop specific training aimed at improving performance according to needs indicated by the reports.
- **Mentoring**: Identify and train staff with strong skills to mentor and assist others in improving performance.
- **Resources**: Productivity reports often highlight resource needs. Supply staff with the equipment and support they need to achieve performance improvement.

NECESSARY INTEGRATION OF THE RESULTS OF DATA ANALYSIS

Integrating the results of data analysis into performance improvement is necessary because attempting performance improvement without data is essentially operating blind. Data should be used not only as the basis for long term strategic planning, but for identifying opportunities for *performance improvement activities* on an ongoing basis. Integration of information includes:

- Identifying issues for tracking.
- Reviewing patterns and trends to determine how they impact care.
- Establishing action plans and desired outcomes based on the need for improvement.
- Providing information to process improvement teams to facilitate change.
- Evaluating systems and processes for follow-up.
- Monitoring specific cases, criteria, critical pathways, and outcomes.

Integrated information assists with case management and decision-making about patient care, as well as improves critical pathways related to clinical performance, staff performance evaluations, credentialing and privileging.

BENEFITS OF INTEGRATING THE RESULTS OF DATA ANALYSIS

The benefits derived from integrating the results of data analysis into the improvement process are:

- Coordination of management/leadership functions provides more efficient planning.
- Evidence-based care decisions increase cost-effectiveness and improve outcomes.
- Duplication of effort is reduced through the sharing of information, increasing the overall efficiency of the organization.
- Staff utilization is more effective.
- Improved accountability allows for better performance assessment.
- Communication among departments/areas within an organization is improved.
- The use of a common database facilitates tracking of patterns and trends.
- Responses can be tailored to the needs of staff, patients, and the organization as a whole.
- Organizational obstacles are dealt with more efficiently because of supporting data.

Performance and Process Improvement

QUALITY IMPROVEMENT PROJECTS

The steps the CPHQ must take for coordination of **quality improvement projects** are:

1. Secure support, resources, and approval from the governing board and key administrative and professional leaders, building support and commitment.
2. Build relationships among staff to facilitate change.
3. Assess the needs of the organization, the climate for change, and the extent of support and resistance in the organization.
4. Produce an internal action plan describing problems that need resolution, development needs, process steps to be completed, responsible staff, and a timeline for completion of tasks.
5. Delineate resource needs, including staffing and training, with a detailed budget outlining the statistical, clerical, and technical needs.
6. Clarify roles and responsibilities organization-wide.
7. Educate staff regarding the mission, vision, values, philosophy of quality management, techniques and tools, benefits, and accreditation and regulatory needs.

Building effectiveness into **quality improvement projects** requires an ongoing commitment at all levels of the organization. The CPHQ oversees these elements:

- Clearly identify leadership roles at all levels in writing.
- Consistently use a common quality language, such as quality management (QM), continuous quality management (CQM), total quality management (TQM).
- Simplify the accountability structure and eliminate redundancy, determining which bodies have ultimate responsibility for decisions and prioritizing, such as a Quality Council.
- Create a flow chart that outlines the quality improvement structure.
- Align organization policies, mission, vision statements, and strategic goals to quality improvement goals.
- Identify organizational functions, including patient care.
- Outline the methodology for performance improvement.
- Establish a structure for periodic reporting and summaries.
- Create interdisciplinary teams.
- Write an implementation plan for organization-wide quality improvement.
- Identify education needs and provide training for teams and leaders.

Establishing Priorities

PRIORITIZING PROCESS IMPROVEMENT ACTIVITIES

Many activities will be identified for process improvement. It is unfeasible to deal with all of them simultaneously, so **prioritize** them for sequential investigation. Defer or ignore single events or those with low impact.

Assemble teams that include upper management and subject matter experts (SME) who are familiar with the needs of the organization. The team decides on which processes they should focus and sets the performance measures.

The team considers which issues require more analysis and looks at existing outcomes that need improvement:

- Risk management and safety violations if the problem is not resolved
- Probability of improved outcomes
- Overall impact on efficiency and delivery of care
- Number of parties involved
- Costs in staff, time, and money
- Relation to mission, vision, and strategic goals
- Frequency and duration of the problem

PRIORITIZATION MATRIX

A **prioritization matrix** determines which item takes precedence, based on pre-selected criteria. The steps for forming a prioritization matrix are:

- Brainstorm to generate a list of problems or options.
- List selection criteria, e.g., cost, patient outcome, and safety.
- Determine the relative value of each criterion and assign weighted points accordingly. For example, each vote for safety is worth 3 points, patient outcome is worth 2 points, and cost is worth 1 point.
- Create a table with enough columns to fit the number of criteria.
- Title the left column "Problems/Options." Title the middle column "Criteria". Title the right column "Total Points."

Team members vote by one of these methods:

- Check marking those criteria that apply
- Using a scale from 1–5, where 1 is the least important and 5 is the most important
- Using a yes/no or + and - system
- Total the scores to rank the priorities

MULTIVOTING

Multivoting is a procedure to prioritize and reach consensus when selecting process improvement activities:

- Review the initial list for redundancies and similarities. Combine like items if the group agrees. Restate the item as agreed by the team.
- Number the remaining items on the list, without prioritizing them.
- Select a voting method, such as colored dots, a point system, or a ranking system. A simple method is one-half plus one (one dot more than half the number of items).
- Vote using the chosen method and tally the votes to determine which items have the most votes.
- Discuss the items that received the most votes.
- Eliminate items with no votes or few votes.
- Repeat the voting and discussion procedure until the list has narrowed. Use voting to prioritize the remaining items.

AFFINITY DIAGRAM

Use an **affinity diagram** to brainstorm and organize **more than 15** ideas, items, or issues into major categories:

Brainstorm to generate a list of ideas. Write each one on a Post-it note or 3x5 card.

Display the Post-its or cards at random on a table or wall.

Sort the ideas into groups, silently and quickly. Find two ideas that go together. Place them to one side. Add to each group until all cards have been either grouped or stand isolated. Discuss each group and agree to a title for each group. If some groups have sub-groups, then create subheadings and move one group under another as a sub-group.

Draw a diagram with the idea at the top, the titles below, and the subheadings beneath.

BRAINSTORMING

Brainstorming is a component of almost all planning and prioritizing activities. Brainstorming generates ideas about problems, process, solutions, or other criteria in a short time frame. Brainstorming may be **structured**, with each person in the group providing an idea in rotation, or **unstructured**, with participants contributing at will. There are 5 primary steps:

1. Establish the purpose of the brainstorming and a time frame.
2. Decide on a structured or unstructured approach.
3. Allow time for general discussion or individual thought.
4. List ideas according to the approach. Write ideas on a white board, flip chart, overhead projector acetate, or computer, so the group can look at the list.
5. Discuss items, clarify, and combine like items as the group agrees.

Ask members to rate or rank items on the list individually. Assign points to each item. Prioritize the list accordingly.

Developing Action Plans

Steps for developing an action plan:

1. Monitor and assess problems for a period of one month, if possible.
2. Prioritize problems.
3. Assign teams to focus on particular problems, based on their knowledge of or participation in the process selected, and their commitment to improvement.
4. Coach each team to write a performance improvement action plan:
5. Systematically identify reasons for variation in a process. Perform a root cause analysis. Identify feasible changes in process.
6. Formulate an action plan that clearly outlines the expected outcomes, steps in the plan, responsibility, timeline, and types of measurements to use for monitoring and evaluation.
7. Conduct a pilot test, after determining the timeframe, sample size, and locations.
8. Analyze data from the pilot test.
9. Modify the action plan, and conduct further pilot testing.
10. Commit resources to the action plan. Involve individuals, departments, and areas involved in the process, and the appropriate leaders.
11. Implement the action plan on a *limited* trial basis, *after* providing training and rescheduling staff.
12. Determine the most effective performance measures.
13. Establish a timeline for *full* implementation.
14. Evaluate the trial implementation and make changes or further analysis, as indicated.
15. Provide clear, detailed communication to all those involved in the process.
16. Incorporate action plans into organizational procedures, and fully implement the action plan.
17. Continue to monitor implementation through performance measures, data collection, surveys, and other feedback from those involved.
18. Monitor and evaluate the impact on patient care, and whether the goals were achieved through changes in process.
19. Document the implementation process and the results.
20. Disseminate the report organization-wide.

ANALYSIS OF PROCESS

Analysis of process currently in use is a critical step in the development of action plans for performance improvement. It involves **aggregation** of data (gathering it together) and **analysis** of each part of the data. The data is used to facilitate change only, not for disciplinary reasons. The purpose of the analysis process is to develop a clear profile of the organization's current level of performance, the stability of current processes, areas of needed improvement, strategies for improving processes, and consistency of design and priorities. The goals of process analysis are:

- **Internal comparison**, which reviews patterns and trends, sentinel events, and upper and lower control limits (guardrails).
- **External comparison** as a reference base of the manner in which others perform similar processes and their outcomes.
- **Standards comparison**, which compares internal data with knowledge-based practice guidelines and regulations.
- **Benchmark comparison**, which may be internal or external, and compares data with benchmark or best practice data.

JURAN QUALITY PLANNING PROCESS

The **Juran quality planning process** is a systematic approach to development of action plans and can be used for strategic plans, quality design, patient safety programs, clinical standards, benchmarking, development of performance measures, and parts of process improvement. It may be used to design new processes, or to modify or redesign previously-existing processes:

- ***Establish the project***: Prioritize, establish teams, and write goals.
- ***Identify customers***: Completely assess the internal and external customers and their needs.
- ***Design or redesign the implementation process***: Describe the current process. Perform a literature review. Identify benchmarks and best practices. Assess customer needs, in light of the latest information available.
- ***Evaluate needs***: Including training; implementation costs in terms of time, staff, and money; resource needs; and expected outcomes.

Performance Improvement Methods

PDCA Pᴇʀfᴏʀmᴀɴᴄᴇ Imᴘʀᴏᴠᴇmᴇɴᴛ Mᴏᴅᴇʟ

Plan-Do-Check-Act (PDCA or Shewhart cycle) is a method of continuous quality improvement. PDCA is simple and understandable; however, it may be difficult to maintain this cycle consistently because of lack of focus and commitment. PDCA is more suited to solving specific problems, rather than organization-wide problems:

- **Plan:** Identify, analyze and define the problem. Set goals and establish a process that coordinates with leadership. Brainstorm extensively. Use Ishikawa fishbone diagrams to identify problematic processes and list current process steps. Collect data and analyze the root cause.
- **Do:** Generate multiple solutions. Select one or more and then implement the first solution on a trial basis.
- **Check:** Gather and analyze data to determine the effectiveness of the first solution. If effective, then continue to *Act*; if not, return to *Plan* and pick a different solution. (*Study* may replace *Check: PDSA.*)
- **Act:** Identify changes that need to be accomplished to fully implement the solution. Adopt the solution and continue to monitor results, while picking another improvement project.

FOCUS Pᴇʀfᴏʀmᴀɴᴄᴇ Imᴘʀᴏᴠᴇmᴇɴᴛ Mᴏᴅᴇʟ

Find, organize, clarify, uncover, and start (**FOCUS**) is a performance improvement model:

- **Find:** Identify a problem by looking at the organization and attempting to determine what isn't working well or what is wrong.
- **Organize:** Identify the people who understand the problem or process and create a team to work on improving performance.
- **Clarify:** Utilize brainstorming techniques, such as Ishikawa fishbone diagrams, to determine what is involved in solving the problem.
- **Uncover:** Analyze the situation to determine the reason the problem has arisen or why a process is unsuccessful.
- **Start:** Determine where to begin the change process.
- FOCUS, by itself, is an incomplete process and is primarily used as a means to identify a problem, rather than a means to find the solution.

FOCUS is usually combined with PDCA (FOCUS-PDCA), so it becomes a 9-step process, but beginning with FOCUS *refines* the problem, resulting in better outcomes.

Aᴄᴄᴇʟᴇʀᴀᴛᴇᴅ Rᴀᴘɪᴅ-Cʏᴄʟᴇ Cʜᴀɴɢᴇ Mᴏᴅᴇʟ

The **accelerated rapid-cycle change approach** is a response to rapid changes in healthcare delivery and radical re-engineering. There are four areas of concern:

- **Models for rapid-cycle change:** The goal is doubling or tripling the rate of quality improvement by modifying and accelerating traditional methods. Teams focus on generating and testing solutions, rather than analysis.
- **Pre-work:** Assigned personnel prepare problem statements, graphic demonstrations of data, flowcharts, and a literature review. Team members are identified.
- **Team creation:** Rapid action teams (RATs, or rapid acceleration, or rapid achievement) are created to facilitate quick change.

- Team meetings and work flow is done over 6 weeks:
  - *Week 1*: Review information. Clarify quality improvement opportunities. Identify key customers, waste, and benchmarks.
  - *Week 2:* Review customer requirements. Perform a cost/benefit analysis of the solution with test data.
  - *Week 3*: Complete the solution's design. Plan its implementation. Conduct pilot tests.
  - *Weeks 4-5:* Test, train, analyze, and make changes as needed.
  - *Week 6:* Implement the solution.

XEROX 10-STEP BENCHMARKING MODEL

Benchmarking is an ongoing process of measuring a practice, service, or product results against their competitors' or industry standards. **Xerox Corporation** developed the **10-step benchmarking model**. The CPHQ needs to know how efficient others' processes are, and search their data for ways to improve the processes. There are four phases in benchmarking: **Planning**, **analysis**, **integration**, and **action**. The 10 steps are:

1. Identify the benchmark targets.
2. Identify similar organizations with which to compare data.
3. Determine and initiate methods of data collection.
4. Evaluate current performance level and deficits.
5. Project a vision of future performance.
6. Communicate findings and reach a group agreement.
7. Recommend changes, based on benchmarking data.
8. Develop specific action plans for objectives.
9. Implement actions and adjust them as necessary, based on monitoring of the process.
10. Update benchmarks based on the latest data.

This basic benchmarking model is often **modified**. It can be shortened to 7 steps, or extended to 11 steps, depending on the needs of the organization. Benchmarking is often used to improve cash flow, as healthcare becomes more competitive, and to compare infection rates.

ERNST AND YOUNG'S 7-STEP "IMPROVE" MODEL

The **Ernst and Young 7-step IMPROVE model** is a simplified model that is effective for teams who are already experienced with quality improvement processes and data collection. The basic steps for the IMPROVE model are:

- **Identify:** Select a problem and evaluate current performance.
- **Measure:** Determine its impact on internal and external customers through evaluation of dates and other information.
- **Prioritize:** Identify all possible causes for the problem and prioritize it.
- **Research:** Assess and evaluate the problem, including a root cause analysis.
- **Outline:** Determine all possible solutions to the problem and develop an action plan to implement appropriate solutions.
- **Validate:** Establish a monitoring system after implementation to validate the effectiveness of a solution.
- **Execute:** Continue to fully implement the solutions and standardize them, while continuing to monitor efficiency.

ORGANIZATIONAL DYNAMICS "FADE" CYCLE PERFORMANCE IMPROVEMENT MODEL

Organizational Dynamics, a consulting firm, developed a four-phase **FADE** performance cycle for quality improvement. The FADE model uses outputs and inputs. The output from one phase serves as the input for the next. The phases are:

1. **Focus:** Hold brainstorming sessions to create a list of problems. Select one problem. Define the problem, analyze its impact completely, and generate a problem statement (output).
2. **Analyze:** Collect baseline data, identify patterns, and gather general information about factors that influence the problem or outcomes. Make charts and diagrams (output), such as Pareto, fishbones, and flowcharts.
3. **Develop:** Generate a list of possible solutions and choose one solution. Create an action plan for implementation (output).
4. **Execute:** Develop support and commitment for the proposed solution through presentations. Put the plan into effect. Monitor the plan's impact to ensure that the plan is effective.

JURAN QUALITY IMPROVEMENT PROCESS (QIP) MODEL

Joseph **Juran's Quality Improvement Process (QIP)** is a four-step model, focusing on quality control. QIP is based on quality planning, control, and improvement. The steps to the QIP process are:

1. **Define:** Organize the project by listing and prioritizing problems, and identifying a team.
2. **Diagnose:** Analyze the problems and then formulate theories related to their root cause. Test theories.
3. **Remediate:** Consider various alternative solutions. Design and implement specific solutions and controls. Address institutional resistance to change. As causes of problems are identified, remediate them, and processes should improve.
4. **Hold:** Evaluate performance and monitor the control system in order to maintain gains.

AHIMA PROCESS IMPROVEMENT MODEL

The **American Health Information Management Association's process improvement model** for performance improvement is a consensus-building method with 11 steps, which are:

1. Create a list of opportunities for improvement through brainstorming and prioritize the list, choosing one on which to focus.
2. Define the project and create the quality improvement team, who will facilitate the improvement process.
3. Analyze problems related to the process.
4. Create a speculative list of causes as a beginning point.
5. Test assumptions.
6. Perform root cause analysis to identify specific causes related to problems.
7. Consider a number of alternative solutions.
8. Design possible solutions and controls.
9. Reach consensus by addressing resistance to change through education, in-service training, and presentations.
10. Implement solutions and controls.
11. Evaluate performance.

SIX SIGMA® PERFORMANCE IMPROVEMENT MODEL

Six Sigma® is a performance improvement model developed by Motorola to improve its business practices and increase its profits. The Six Sigma® model has been adapted to many types of businesses, including healthcare. Six Sigma® is a **data-driven** performance model that aims to eliminate "defects" in processes that involve products or services. The goal is to achieve Six Sigma, meaning no more than **3.4 defects** in every **1 million opportunities**. The focus is on continuous improvement, with the customer's perception as key, so that the customer defines that which is "critical to quality" (**CTQ**). Two different types of improvement projects may be employed: **DMAIC** (define, measure, analyze, improve, control) for *existing* processes or products that need improvement and **DMADV** (define, measure, analyze, design, verify) for development of *new*, high-quality processes or products. Both DMAIC and DMADV utilize trained personnel to execute the plans. Six Sigma® personnel have martial arts titles: Green belts and black belts execute programs, and master black belts supervise programs.

DMAIC TYPE OF SIX SIGMA® PERFORMANCE IMPROVEMENT PROJECT

The first project type for Six Sigma® is **DMAIC** (define, measure, analyze, improve, control), which is used when existing healthcare processes or products need quality improvement:

- **Define** costs and benefits that will be achieved when the changes are instituted. Develop a list of customer needs, based on complaints and requests.
- **Measure** input, process, and output. Collect baseline data. Perform a cost analysis. Calculate the sigma rating.
- **Analyze** root or other causes of current defects. Use data to confirm analysis. Uncover steps in processes that are counterproductive.
- **Improve** by creating potential solutions. Develop and pilot plans. Measure the results. Determine the cost savings and other benefits to customers.
- **Control** the work processes by standardizing them. Monitor the system by linking performance measures to a balanced scorecard. Create processes for updating procedures, disseminating reports, and recommending future processes.

LEAN-SIX SIGMA® PERFORMANCE IMPROVEMENT MODEL

Lean-Six Sigma® is a performance improvement model that combines Six Sigma® with concepts of "lean" thinking by focusing process improvement on strategic goals, rather than on a project-by-project basis. A Lean-Six program is driven by strong senior leadership, who outline long-term goals and strategies to employees. Physicians are an important part of the Lean-Six process, and must be included and engaged. The basis of Lean-Six is to *reduce errors and waste* within the organization through *continuous learning* and *rapid change*. Lean-Six has four characteristics:

- Long-term goals with strategies in place for -1 to 3-year periods.
- Performance improvement is the underlying belief system.
- Cost reduction through quality increase, supported by statistics evaluating the cost of inefficiency.
- Incorporation of improvement methodology, such as DMAIC, PDCA, or other methods.

NATIONAL AND INTERNATIONAL QUALITY MODELS

There is an increasing need for both **national and international excellence/quality models**, so that best practices and standardizations can be shared. Existing models include:

- Joint Commission Standards for Improvement of Organizational performance, where voluntary compliance leads to accreditation
- The National Committee for Quality Assurance (NCQA) management improvement process
- Baldrige Award Criteria for Process Management and Results, an evaluation process providing excellent performance assessment
- International Standards Organization (ISO) standard for quality management (9001:2000); requires a strategic approach to process improvement through quality planning and supportive data
- United States Federal Quality Improvement Programs, which help organizations remain in compliance with these complex Federal mandates regarding Medicare:
  - o Healthcare Quality Improvement Program (HCQIP)
  - o Quality Improvement Organization (QIO) projects
  - o Quality Improvement System for Managed Care (QISMC)

Healthcare facilities participate in these models to obtain accreditation, comply with Medicare or other Federal program regulations, gain feedback, or gain prestige.

Budget Management

DEPARTMENTAL BUDGETS

DEVELOPING AND MANAGING DEPARTMENTAL BUDGETS

Once the departmental budget is developed and established, **budget management** must occur on an ongoing basis to ensure that financial targets are met in relation to strategic goals. Management includes:

- *Accountability*: The budget team should include managers and directors who expect excellence.
- *Controlling expenses*: This is especially important for departments that do not produce income directly.
- *Monitoring costs in relation to best practice benchmarks:* One goal of budget management is to strive to match benchmarks.
- *Developing corrective action plans*: Any variances in the budget should be accounted for within a week and corrective actions taken.
- *Using a balanced scorecard*: Various measurements, both quantitative and qualitative, are used to manage cost containment strategies.
- *Recognizing quality*: Rewards for achieving benchmarks should be built in to the budgeting process. In some cases, this may be a bonus payout.

UNDERSTANDING OF FINANCIAL MANAGEMENT

Financial management is a part of strategic planning, in which the department demonstrates how its resources will be allocated, usually for a one-year period. Financial management includes: Developing and assigning budget items; monitoring expenditures; analysis; and reporting. Sound financial management is based on the best utilization of costs in relation to revenues and outcomes. Objectives of financial management include:

- Developing a quantitative record of plans
- Allowing for evaluation of financial performance
- Controlling costs
- Providing information to increase cost awareness

The budget must be linked to **daily operations** and integrated with strategic vision, mission, goals, and objectives. Those with vested interests in the budget should participate in its planning. **Monitoring** should be ongoing to allow for feedback and modifications as necessary.

TYPES OF BUDGETS

A **departmental budget** is part of a larger organizational budget. The CPHQ must understand the different types of budgets used in healthcare, in order to participate in financial management:

- *Operating budget*: The operating budget has 3 elements: Statistics, expenses, and revenue. It is used for daily operations, and includes general expenses, such as salaries, education, insurance, maintenance, depreciation, debts, and profit.
- *Capital budget*: The capital budget determines which capital projects (such as remodeling, repairing, and purchasing of equipment or buildings) will be allocated funding for the year. These capital expenditures are usually based on cost-benefit analysis and prioritization of needs.

- ***Cash balance budget:*** The cash balance budget projects cash balances for a specific future time period, including all operating and capital budget items.
- ***Master budget:*** The master budget combines operating, capital, and cash balance budgets, and any specialized or area-specific budgets.

DIFFERENT APPROACHES TO DEPARTMENTAL BUDGETS

Most **departmental budgets** are operational, but a number of different approaches can be used:

- ***Fixed/forecast:*** Revenue and expenses are forecast for the entire budget period and budget items are fixed.
- ***Flexible:*** Estimates are made regarding anticipated changes in revenue and expenses, and both fixed and variable costs are identified.
- ***Zero-based:*** All cost centers are re-evaluated each budget period to determine if they should be funded or eliminated, partially or completely.
- ***Responsibility center:*** Budgeting is a cost center (department) or centers with one person holding overall responsibility.
- ***Program:*** Organizational programs are identified, and revenues and costs for each program are budgeted.
- ***Appropriations:*** Government funds are requested and dispersed through appropriations.
- ***Continuous/rolling:*** Periodic updates to the budget, including revenues, costs, and volume, are done prior to the next budget cycle.

ACTIVITY-BASED COSTING (ABC) SYSTEM

The **activity-based costing (ABC)** system is an accounting system that focuses on the ***costs of resources*** necessary for a process or service. There are some differences between ABC and traditional accounting, which is a cash-based system where the bookkeeper enters revenues when they are received and expenses when they are paid, so that revenues and expenses are not necessarily related. By contrast, ABC is an accrual system, where the bookkeeper enters revenues when they are earned and expenses as they are incurred, so that revenues and expenses are more closely tied. The basic formula for ABC is to divide the ***total output*** into ***total cost*** to arrive at a ***unit cost***. The general steps to ABC are:

- Identify activities involved in processes and outputs
- Calculate cost of resources for activities, including direct costs, indirect costs, and administrative (general overhead) costs
- Identify all outputs related to activities and utilization of resources
- Allocate costs of activities to outputs; cost drivers are costs of resources related to activities

FINANCIAL COSTS RELATED TO QUALITY MANAGEMENT

Performance improvement is not without costs, and these must be considered carefully when doing a cost analysis. Financial **costs related to quality** management include:

Error-free costs, which are the costs of all processes, services, equipment, time, materials, and staffing necessary to provide a product or process that is without error from its outset. A process that is error-free is relatively stable in terms of pre-established guidelines.

Cost of quality (COQ) includes costs associated with identifying and correcting errors, making errors, defects or failures in processes and planning, and costs of poor quality (COPQ). **Conformance costs** are those costs related to preventing errors, such as monitoring and evaluation. This may include education, maintenance, pilot testing, and analysis. ***Nonconformance costs*** are those related to errors, failures, and defects. These include adverse events (such as infections), poor patient access due to staff shortages, appointment and surgery cancellations, lost time, duplications of service, and malpractice fines.

JUSTIFYING EXPENDITURES USING A COST-BENEFIT ANALYSIS

A **cost-benefit analysis** uses the average cost of an event and the cost of an intervention to demonstrate savings. For example: According to the CDC, a surgical site infection caused by *Staphylococcus aureus* results in an average of 12 additional days of hospitalization and costs $27,000. (In actuality, the cost varies widely from one institution to another, so use local data if it benefits the institution's case.) If an institution averages 10 surgical site infections annually, the cost is 10 x $27,000 = **$270,000** annually.

If the proposed interventions include:

- New software for surveillance ($10,000)
- An additional staff person ($65,000 salary + $15,000 benefits)
- Increased staff education, including materials ($2000)
- Then the total intervention cost would be $10,000 + $65,000 +$15,000 + $2000 = **$92,000.00**

If the goal were to decrease infections by 50%, to 5 infections per year, the savings would be 5 x $27,000 = **$135,000**

Subtract the intervention cost from the savings to obtain the annual cost benefit: $135,000 - $92,000 = **$43,000**

A **cost-effective analysis** measures the effectiveness of an intervention rather than its monetary savings. For example:

Each year, 2 million nosocomial infections result in 90,000 deaths and $6.7 billion in additional health costs. From that perspective, decreasing infections should reduce costs, but there are human savings in suffering as well, and it is difficult to place a dollar value on that. If each infection adds about 12 days to hospitalization, then a reduction in infection by 5 days would be calculated as: 5 x 12 = 60 fewer patient infection days.

Efficacy studies compare a series of cost-benefit analyses to determine the intervention with the best cost-benefit. Efficacy studies can also be used for ***process or product evaluation.*** For example:

A study is conducted to determine the infection rates of four different types of catheters. The catheter type that results in the fewest infections thus saves the most money and infection days.

Incremental cost-effectiveness ratio is the difference between a cost change and an outcome change.

JUSTIFYING EXPENDITURES USING A COST-UTILITY ANALYSIS

Cost-utility analysis (CUA) is essentially a sub-type of cost-effective analysis, but CUA is more complex and its results are more difficult to quantify and use to justify expense. Cost-utility analysis measures the benefit of an intervention to society in general, such as decreasing teenage pregnancies. Often, the standards used to quantify CUA are somewhat subjective. CUA compares a variety of outcomes (e.g., increased life expectancy and decreased suffering) in relation to the **quality-adjusted-life-year** (QALY). A health condition is assigned a number on a scale—referred to as its ***utility***—in which 1 represents normal health and 0 represents death. When calculating outcomes with CUA, an intervention is evaluated on whether or not it increases the utility score, and thereby increases life expectancy or improves life circumstances by X number of years. Thus, the CUA results are not expressed as monetary values, but rather as societal values.

JUSTIFYING EXPENDITURES USING A COST ALLOCATION

One type of cost analysis involves **cost allocation.** With almost all expenditures, there are ***direct*** costs and ***indirect*** costs. For example, the salary of a team leader is a direct cost. Indirect costs are those related to Accounting and Human Resources. To determine cost allocation, the CPHQ must use line item budget format. List each item with its unit cost or cost per unit of service. Determine direct costs and indirect costs. Generally, direct costs benefit just one department or service, while indirect costs are shared costs, such as the cost of custodial services. Thus, a percentage of the indirect cost is allocated to a department based on its utilization.

For example: If team leaders represent 5% of the total employees, then 5% of indirect employee costs would be allocated to this line item. Remember, there are many departments and services involved in indirect costs. To arrive at *a **true unit cost***, account for all of these costs.

Establish Teams, Roles, Responsibilities and Scope

PERFORMANCE IMPROVEMENT TEAM

A **performance improvement team** is a group of people working together to achieve a goal, like writing a clinical action plan. Performance improvement activities almost always involve a team or teams of staff because of the complexity of healthcare organizations. Rarely is one department solely responsible for outcomes, except in very specialized work. **Tracer methodology** is a method that looks at the continuum of care a patient receives from admission to post-discharge. When determining the composition of the performance improvement team, use tracer methodology to ensure there is at least one representative from all groups that participate in patient care on the team. Teamwork requires a considerable time and training commitment. Performance improvement initiatives require teams to:

- Improve outcomes through a common purpose
- Utilize staff expertise
- Contribute various perspectives
- Facilitate a participative management style
- Improve acceptance of processes that impact work practice
- Manage complexity, where many participants are involved
- Increase organization-wide acceptance of change
- Combat resistance to change

Advantages of developing performance improvement teams include:

- *Individual***:** Team members have the opportunity to develop new skills, share their expertise, utilize their creativity, increase their personal autonomy, influence decisions, and improve their job satisfaction. Working in teams often increases the team members' respect for other disciplines and members.
- *Administrative***:** The organization's administration benefits when it has increased flexibility to facilitate, rather than direct. Delegating performance improvement to teams means administrators have fewer time constraints, increased staff support, better utilization of skills, and improved productivity. Utilizing teams frees administrators from many time-consuming tasks, allowing for better overall management.
- *Organization-wide***:** The organization benefits by more continuity, customer satisfaction, cost efficiency, improved productivity, more efficient accountability, decreased staff turnover, and an improved ability to deal with staff turnover. Teams benefit the entire organization because they are more suited to dealing with complexity than individuals.

TEAM STRUCTURE

The appropriate **team structure** is very important in performance improvement because creating a team does not, in itself, assure teamwork. The team must be comprised of individuals whose skills complement each other and who have a shared purpose, because outcomes depend on the collaborative efforts of the group, rather than individuals within the group. Accordingly, the collective team is accountable for outcomes, rather than individuals. When creating teams, consider these important elements:

- **Size:** Teams with less than 10 members are most effective.
- **Skills:** Team members should have complementary skills that encompass the technical, problem solving, decision-making, and interpersonal aspects of the problem.

- **Performance goals:** Allow teams a degree of autonomy to produce action plans for performance improvement, based on strategic goals and objectives.
- **Unified approach:** Create the teams according to the model of performance improvement chosen but allow them some flexibility in working together.
- **Accountability:** Make the team members collectively accountable, rather than individually accountable.

CROSS-FUNCTIONAL TEAMS

Cross-functional teams are sometimes called ***interdisciplinary***. Cross-functional teams are comprised of individuals with various skill levels or from different disciplines, who work together to accomplish one or more functions. An ***ad hoc team*** operates for a short time to accomplish specific goals. A ***permanent team*** is a regular part of continuous performance improvement. Cross-functional teams are particularly useful when it is required to:

- Develop new processes.
- Implement organization-wide performance changes or technology.
- Control costs and increase the cost-benefit ratio.
- Deal with problems or performance activities that cross disciplines.
- Access a broad range of expertise and skills.

To ensure the success of performance improvement activities:

- Select team members with the correct mix of abilities.
- Clearly outline the roles for the team members.
- List the expected outcomes.
- Provide adequate training to assist cross-functional team members in working together as a unit.

SELF-DIRECTED WORK TEAMS

Self-directed work teams are groups of individuals working together to achieve a common goal, such as improving a process or producing a product. While the members may be trained cross-functionally, they usually have individual functions within the group. Usually, the teams have an assigned task or tasks for which they are accountable, but have the authority to manage the functions on their own, and make decisions without the direction of the administration. As with other types of teams, self-directed work teams may be ***ad hoc*** or ***permanent***. Their degree of autonomy varies from one organization to another. Self-directed work teams may do the following:

- Plan and establish priorities
- Organize and manage budgets
- Manage work schedules and assignments
- Engage in problem-solving activities and make corrections
- Monitor and evaluate performance
- Coordinate with other teams or individuals
- Choose or hire team members

PERFORMANCE OVERSIGHT GROUP

The **performance oversight group** is often referred to as the quality council, steering council, or quality management committee. The governing board establishes the performance oversight group to coordinate all **performance improvement activities**. The group is usually drawn from administrative leaders, medical staff, and key personnel in various departments. The chairperson of the group is usually appointed by the President or Chief Executive Officer of the organization, and is approved by the medical staff and governing board. Part of the role of the facilitator is to:

- Inform the governing board of the need for the group.
- Cost the group's activities.
- Develop a preliminary list of group responsibilities.
- Match those responsibilities with the skills, knowledge, work roles, and vision of potential group members.
- Schedule regular meetings for the group, ranging from twice monthly to 10 times yearly.
- Report the group's activities regularly to the governing board.
- Document the group's performance improvement activities.
- Maintain confidentiality of patient and practitioner information, in accordance with HIPAA regulations.

The **performance oversight group** has tremendous influence over the success of a performance improvement plan, so potential group members must be aware of their **responsibilities** and willing to **participate**. Disseminate preliminary information about performance improvement at meetings held to discuss the issues. The responsibilities of the performance oversight group are to:

- Develop, modify, and approve the performance improvement plan
- Establish priorities for initiatives, based on patient impact, data, and organizational objectives
- Select the types of teams needed, establish teams, and supervise them
- Plan methodologies to support action plans
- Review aggregate data, measurements of performance, and periodic summaries from teams
- Establish a confidential peer review policy
- Establish educational and training programs as needed
- Supervise a budget and make budgetary recommendations
- Evaluate the effectiveness of performance activities
- Provide summaries of achievement activities and progress toward goals

ROLES WITHIN A PERFORMANCE IMPROVEMENT TEAM

There are a number of **key roles** within a performance improvement team, and selecting the best-suited candidate to fill each role greatly influences the effectiveness of the team. The key roles are:

- **Facilitator** (Master Black belt in Six Sigma®): The facilitator is not a member of the team, but rather consults with or coaches the team members, helps to build team skills, and keeps the team focused. The facilitator may: Provide training, assist the team leader or team members, receive input from team members, evaluate consensus, provide feedback, and summarize outcomes.
- **Team leader** (Black belt in Six Sigma®): This team leader is a member of the team who provides direction, but is not individually responsible for decision-making, or the overall effectiveness of the team's efforts. Often, team leaders are middle managers that coach, rather than direct, members of the team. The team leader may: Prepare and conduct meetings; assign activities; evaluate progress; coordinate with other teams; communicate with the facilitator; and document meetings and activities.

- **Team member** (Green belt in Six Sigma®): The team member is a critical part of the team because this person does much of the actual hands-on activities related to team responsibilities. The team member: Attends all meetings; provides input for the agenda; assists the team leader; shares expertise; communicates with other team members; completes specific assignments; proposes projects; measures; collects data; and recommends actions.
- **Secretary/recorder:** The Secretary is responsible for keeping minutes and creating other reports or documents as needed by the team. This position may become the responsibility of one person or may be done on a rotating basis by various team members. Careful documentation and reporting are a necessary function of teams, so that their progress can be evaluated and reports disseminated to management.
- **Timekeeper:** The timekeeper monitors the time spent in meetings and keeps people on track, so that meeting times are well spent, and do not exceed scheduled times. This position is often rotated among team members.
- **Sponsor (champion):** The sponsor may be the quality council as a whole, or a key leader with an interest in the particular activities of a team. The sponsor is not involved in the day-to-day activity of the group, but receives regular reports regarding the team's activities. The sponsor reviews the team's efforts and may provide guidance or direction. The sponsor maintains overall responsibility and accountability for the team effort, and has a primary role in the selection of projects and other members of the team. The sponsor ensures that all interested parties are informed, monitors decisions and activities, and has the authority to implement changes.

CHAMPIONS VS. PROCESS OWNERS

Champions are those individuals with a particular passion for or interest in the activities of a performance improvement team and are often instrumental in the creation and formation of the teams themselves, choosing the basic function of the team and the team members. Because members of organizations very often resist change, the champion has a pivotal role in providing leadership.

- The *process champion* (also called a *sponsor*) is often a member of upper management, who has the authority to make decisions, and the ability to communicate with top management and the governing board.
- Champions can exist at different levels, so there may be *clinical champions* or *patient safety champions* — individuals who have made an effort to be informed and to promote performance improvement.
- *Process owners*, on the other hand, are usually the team leaders, who are actively involved in supervising and/or carrying out the functions and activities of the team. Process owners are often key managers with knowledge and commitment to improvement.

TEAMBUILDING

Leading, facilitating, and participating in performance improvement teams requires a thorough understanding of **team-building dynamics**:

- *Initial interactions:* The time when members define their roles and develop relationships, which determines if they are comfortable in the group.
- *Power issues:* The members observe the leader and determine who controls the meeting and how control is exercised; they begin to form alliances.
- *Organizing:* Methods to achieve work are clarified and team members begin to work together, gaining respect for each other's contributions and working toward a common goal.

130

- **Team identification:** Interactions become less formal as members develop rapport, so members are more willing to help and support each other to achieve goals.
- **Excellence:** The team achieves success through a combination of good leadership, committed team members, clear goals, high standards, external recognition, a spirit of collaboration, and a shared commitment to the process.

LEADING MEETINGS

Good **techniques for leading meetings** include:

- **Scheduling:** Review the work schedules of those involved. Find the most convenient time for all attendees. Choose a place convenient and conducive to working together. Meeting rooms must have a round table to facilitate an equal exchange of ideas, or room to sit in a circle. Order computers, overhead projectors, whiteboards, a tape recorder, and any other necessary equipment.
- **Preparation:** Prepare a detailed agenda with a list of items for discussion and approximate time limit for each. E-mail the minutes from the last meeting to attendees.
- **Conduction:** Introduce each item on the agenda and solicit input from all group members. Assign tasks to individual members based on their interest and part in the process. Summarize input and begin a tentative future agenda. Announce the time and place of the next meeting.
- **Observation:** Watch the interactions of team members, including verbal and non-verbal communication, and respond.

PREPARING A TEAM CONTRACT

Many problems that arise with teams are avoidable if the team members reach a consensus about their expectations before group work begins. Complete a **team contract** at the initial meeting. All members must participate. Team contracts include these sections:

- **Roles:** Delineate the specific responsibilities of each team member, including the leader.
- **Discussion:** Decide if meetings will be agenda-driven, follow Robert's rules, or open discussion.
- **Time:** State the amount of time that members are expected to commit to team activities, including attending meetings.
- **Conduct:** Clarify acceptable parameters for behavior, including those for the individuals and the group.
- **Conflict resolution:** Agree on triggers for conflict resolution and methods.
- **Reports:** List the types of reports, timeline, and responsibility for preparing the reports.
- **Consequences:** Clearly state the penalty for failure to follow the contract.

DELEGATING TASKS

Effective leaders **delegate** work. Leaders who take on too much of the workload cripple themselves. Failure to delegate shows an inherent distrust in team members. To delegate effectively:

- Assess the skills and available time of the team members; determine if a task is suitable for an individual.
- Assign tasks with clear instructions and a timeline; explain objectives and expectations.
- Ensure tasks are completed properly and on time by monitoring progress, but not by micromanaging.
- Review the final results and record outcomes.

Mentor, monitor, and provide feedback and intervention as necessary during this process, because the leader is ultimately responsible for the delegated work. While delegated tasks may not always be completed successfully, they represent learning opportunities for staff.

REFRAINING FROM DELEGATING TASKS

Delegation of tasks in central to working in teams, but the leader must decide which tasks to perform **personally**. Not every task can be delegated. Retain tasks related to strategic planning and management:

- **Leadership**: Regardless of one's leadership style, ultimate authority and responsibility for teamwork is retained by the leader. Shared leadership duties lead to confusion and resentment on the part of team members.
- **Monitoring**: Control the process through effective monitoring to ensure all tasks are completed ȯn time.
- **Discipline**: Deal with misconduct privately; do not discuss it with the group.
- **Strategic goals and planning**: The leader is responsible for keeping the goals in mind and working toward the organizational vision.
- **Communication**: Keep all members informed. Be available for consultation.
- **Outcomes assessment**: Direct the final performance review; debrief and disband personally.

MANAGEMENT'S LINES OF AUTHORITY AND ACCOUNTABILITY

The Joint Commission has established leadership standards that apply to healthcare organizations and help to establish management's **lines of authority and accountability.** Under these standards, leadership comprises the governing body, the Chief Executive Officer, senior managers, department leaders, leaders (both elected and appointed) of staff or departments, the Nursing Executive, and other nurse leaders. The governing body is ultimately responsible for all patient care rendered by all types of practitioners (physicians, nurses, laboratory staff, and support staff) within and under the jurisdiction of the organization. The governing body must clearly outline the lines of authority and accountability for others in management positions. Each level of management must establish **performance standards** and **performance measurements**, so that accountability becomes transparent, and is based on data that can be used to drive changes when needed, to bring about improved outcomes.

> **Review Video: The Joint Commission Core Principles**
> Visit mometrix.com/academy and enter code: 676427

Performance Improvement Plan Development

DEVELOPING PERFORMANCE IMPROVEMENT PLANS

To **develop a performance improvement plan**, follow these steps:

1. **Design the process:** Choose an approach that focuses on quality planning, control, and improvement. Assemble a team. Establish a process based on data. Identify customers. Assess the organization's ability to implement a plan. Include training needs and resources in the initial design.

2. **Design the plan**: Plan strategically for organization-wide participation and collaborative activities, which may be department or discipline-specific, or interdisciplinary. Make the plan consistent with the organization's vision and mission statements, and its goals and objectives. Include performance expectations and measurements.
3. **Plan for implementation**: Write the plan, including: A definition of quality; standards of care; guidelines for patient safety; benchmarks; and outcome measurements. Educate leadership and staff.

The CPHQ must resolve these issues to develop a **performance improvement plan:**

- **Leadership roles**: Delineate the roles of the key leaders *in writing*, beginning at the highest level (such as the Chief Executive Officer), so that their responsibilities are clear.
- **Terminology related to quality**: Use *consistent terminology* in all documents and activities. Decide whether to refer to quality management (QM), quality resource management (QRM), continuous quality improvement (CQI) or some other acronym.
- **Accountability structure**: Determine who will sit on the quality council. Its members set priorities regarding staff time, finances, and resources, and ensure accountability. The quality council should be one structure, which may require the integration of existing bodies or the creation of a new entity. The quality council oversees the plan, reports to the governing board, and communicates with leaders at all levels.

VITAL PAPERWORK

As part of the process of developing a performance improvement plan, the CPHQ should:

- **Create a flow chart**: Include the complete organizational structure, with all the participating councils, teams, and lines of authority and communication. Provide a copy for all team members.
- **Integrate policies, statements, and plans**: Update documentation across the organization, so that all use the same terminology (e.g., customers or consumers, public or non-staff). Make a consistent glossary of definitions.
- **Link goals with performance improvement activities**: All performance activities must reference the organization's specific strategic goals or objectives and its mission and vision statements. If there is a disparity, then either the vision and mission statements must be adjusted, or the focus of the improvement activities must be changed. The mission and vision statements are central to quality healthcare planning. Plan all activities with the intention of meeting established goals and objectives.

TEAM REPORTING AND STRUCTURES

A performance improvement plan requires the CPHQ to:

- **Establish a reporting structure and calendar**: Performance improvement activities are usually reported on a monthly basis or another regular, frequent schedule. Distribute a detailed written report *and* present a synopsis at team and management meetings. Remind the directors and managers to disseminate the monthly report through staff meetings. Post a calendar, which clearly indicates a proposed timeline for improvements, and lists regular meetings times.
- **Determine the team structures**: A number of different teams may be necessary, depending on the model selected. Assign the teams very specific functions, such as patient assessment, clinical improvement, and operations improvement. Determine which teams should be interdisciplinary, which teams should be department-specific, and who should be included.

WRITING PERFORMANCE IMPROVEMENT PLANS

Document every performance improvement plan in **writing**. Tailor the written plan to its *purpose*. It may be brief if it is intended primarily as a teaching tool to guide staff, but if it is intended as a tool for implementation, it must be a comprehensive document that outlines in detail all of the different aspects of the performance improvement plan. A detailed plan must include a:

- Statement of commitment.
- Clear outline of authority and responsibility.
- Explanation of the infrastructure.
- Outline of the flow of information.

The organization may require a written plan for its **state licensure** or participation in **federal plans**. Obtain a copy of the specific state and federal requirements, and ensure the plan corresponds to them exactly. The goals and objective of a quality plan must clearly relate to the organization's overall strategic goals and objectives. Outline the structure and design of leadership and teams and delineate their responsibilities. Get approvals from all interested parties and keep the originals on file with the document.

ADDRESSING EDUCATIONAL NEEDS AND TEAM TRAINING

A performance improvement plan must:

- ***Identify the specific educational needs of leaders and staff:*** Decide who requires education. State the educational needs of each group of participants, and what the organization can appropriately provide. List the means for providing this education. For example, an organization can provide on-site computer training during regular work hours, but staff must renew their CPR and First Aid certification off-site, in their own time, through an independent third-party provider, like Red Cross. Create an executive summary and detailed plan for all those in leadership positions, beginning with the governing board, so they thoroughly understand the performance improvement plan, its data collection, measurement, and analysis.
- ***Plan for training teams:*** Relate general training to team structure, team functions, and team leadership. Ensure the individual team members get training for their specific roles, so teams work consistently.

FUNCTIONS AND MODEL

Functions are the specialized activities of a system. Functions include not only patient care, but also governance, management, and support. If function is the focus, rather than individual departments, it integrates services and makes patient care the priority, rather than the departmental processes themselves. Identify functions by analyzing patient tracers, performance measures, cost data, reviews, and claims data.

Model (or methodology): The guide for a performance improvement plan, such as FOCUS, PDCA, 10-Step Benchmarking, QIP, or Six Sigma. Review all models and pick the one that best meets the needs of the organization *and* will be accepted by all interested parties. Part of one's decision relates to available resources and the degree of commitment the organization has to performance improvement.

DEMONSTRATING THE FINANCIAL BENEFITS OF A QUALITY PROGRAM

A quality performance improvement plan should not only improve functions (including patient care) but must show a **financial benefit** to the organization if it is to gain support of the governing board. Complete a cost-benefit analysis to demonstrate potential savings or income for each aspect of the action plan. For example, if bar coding will be used to decrease medication errors, thereby reducing complications and shortening hospital stay, then potential savings exist. Provide specific, measurable goals in the improvement plan to facilitate calculation of financial benefits. As the plan is implemented, include a financial benefit section in the monthly written report, because this provides tangible evidence of the plan's success. Summarize the financial benefits in graphs and charts, because a visual demonstration is a more effective way to communicate than text alone.

Tools and Techniques

EVENTS AND CAUSAL FACTORS CHART

The **events and causal factors analysis (E&CF)** chart is a combination of the flow chart and affinity diagram. E&CF lists the **sequential steps** in a process or occurrence and the **conditions affecting each step**. E&CF is useful in root cause analysis and to analyze best practices. The steps for E&CF are:

1. List the name of the process or occurrence in a box on the right (as in a flow chart).
2. List the steps in the process in boxes from right to left (as in a cause-effect diagram), linked with arrows pointing to the process box on the right.
3. Under each event box, place an arrow pointing downward and list all possible factors that contributed to the occurrence at that step through repeatedly asking "Why?" (As in an affinity diagram).
4. Discuss and reach group consensus about root causes to determine actions for performance improvement or (if used to analyze best practices) to ensure a process can be replicated.

STORYBOARDS

A **storyboard** is a visual representation of the **actions of a team**, including data analysis and decisions, during the performance improvement process. It is usually done on a firm poster board, around 3 to 4 feet square. A storyboard looks somewhat like a giant flow chart, with arrows or lines connecting one piece of information to the next. A storyboard includes a wide variety of information:

- Charts
- Diagrams
- Pictures
- Text
- Illustrations
- Statistics

Because the storyboard is meant to provide easy access to information about team activities, keep text minimal.

GANTT CHARTS

A **Gantt chart** is a bar chart with a horizontal time scale used to:

- Develop improvement projects
- Manage schedules
- Estimate time needed to complete tasks

It is a visual representation of the beginning and end time points when different steps in a process should be completed. Gantt charts are available in project management software programs, Excel, and SmartDraw. Create a Gantt chart *after* initial brainstorming, to outline a *timeline* and *action plans*:

- List the name of the process in the header.
- Create a horizontal chart with the timeline of days, weeks, or months (as appropriate for process) across the top.
- List tasks vertically on the left of the chart.

- Draw horizontal lines or bars from the expected beginning point to the expected end point for each task. Color-code task bars to indicate which individual or team is responsible for completing the task.

TASK LISTS

A **task list** is a simple but essential tool for organizing and developing plans. It **assigns responsibility** and helps individuals and teams stay within a **scheduled time frame**:

- Brainstorm to identify and discuss necessary tasks or steps in a process.
- Create a complete master list of tasks and steps.
- Assign responsibility for each task and step to an individual team member.
- Provide a timeframe during which the task or step must be completed.
- Create a task list in chart form, with 4 columns:
  - (Left) Task or step
  - (2nd) Individual responsible for completing task or step
  - (3rd) Due date for completion
  - (Right) Date the task or step is completed
- Update the list as tasks are completed. Share the revised task list with team members, so they can evaluate progress and identify tasks that have not been completed.

DELPHI TECHNIQUE

The **Delphi technique** is a method of consensus building that operates with the idea that, over time and with guidance, people will compromise and move toward similar opinions. This technique can be used to manipulate people's opinions. There are two different Delphi methods:

- **Method I:** A facilitator leads the group. Each member expresses an opinion, and then the facilitator challenges or questions these opinions, sometimes intimidating people into changing their positions, and other times facilitating a better exchange of ideas.
- **Method II:** A questionnaire or listing of options is given to each member so he/she can express an anonymous opinion (before, during, or after meetings). A facilitator or team leader then revises the questionnaire or listing of options, based on the responses, and circulates it again until consensus is reached. Discussion to review results takes place at team meetings.

Evaluation

EVALUATING PERFORMANCE IMPROVEMENT MODELS

A number of different **performance improvement models** have been developed over the years. Evaluating and applying these models are part of strategic management and quality healthcare. Some medical organizations use a single approach, but many combine models in various ways in order to meet their specific needs. Those in leadership roles must understand how these models can facilitate change, so that they choose elements that are appropriate for the needs of their organization and to those who will work with the model. All the various models share some like elements:

- The models focus on **continuous improvement** and are planned, systematic, collaborative, and apply to the entire organization
- They all focus on identifying problems, collecting data, assessing current performance, instituting actions for change, assessing changes, team development, and use of data
- In order for any model or eclectic elements from different models to be effective, there must be **cooperation** and **consensus** across the organization.

MONITORING PROJECT TIMELINESS AND DELIVERABLES

Measuring and monitoring of a project are ongoing procedures that evaluate progress toward objectives and indicate any deviations so that corrections can be made. Activities on the timeline should be assessed to determine if they are on schedule, ahead of schedule, or behind schedule. Risks should be assessed and managed. Changes should be assessed through integrated change control and all change requests documented as well as their approval or rejection. Quality control measurements should be carried out and any defects noted and corrected. Performance of team members should be monitored. Any changes in the scope of a project should be noted and the project plan updated. Performance reports should be completed as scheduled and disseminated to the proper individuals or agencies. A Gantt chart, which is a bar chart with a horizontal time scale that presents a visual representation of the beginning and end points of time for when different steps in a process, may be used to develop and manage the timeline.

MONITORING CONSULTANTS

Many organizations hire **consultants** to facilitate or lead teams or to provide specific services for performance improvement. The CPHQ selects a consultant based on networking, recommendations, advertising, references, telephone interviews, presentations, personal interviews, and proposals. The CPHQ must select the correct consultant, to ensure that:

- Quality and patient safety are not compromised.
- The goals, needs, and budget of the project are met.

The **duties** of the CPHQ are to:

- Make a clear, itemized list of goals for the project.
- Provide an organizational chart to the consultant, clearly defining the lines of authority in relationship to the consultant.
- Create an itemized job description for the consultant.
- Specify time frames and deadlines in the consulting contract.
- Include confidentiality agreements and specific work requirements in the contract.

Once the consultant is hired, the CPHQ **supervises** the consultant's activities, to ensure that the consultant adheres to the job description and provides valued service to the organization.

EVALUATION OF TEAM PERFORMANCE THROUGH PERFORMANCE MEASURES

Evaluation of team performance is a necessary part of performance improvement because of the need for efficient and effective teamwork. Teams are evaluated in three areas of performance:

1. *Completion of assigned tasks*: This includes adhering to timelines, completing the task properly, and producing reports as required.
2. *Ability of the group to work together and reach consensus*: A team must meet regularly, work effectively, and arrive at decisions with minimal conflict.
3. *Effectiveness of the individual team members*: Team members must assume responsibility for completing their parts of tasks and cooperate with others in the group.

Consider each of these elements when developing performance measures for each step in a process to determine if the group is effective.

POOR TEAM PERFORMANCE INDICATORS

When analyzing data for **evaluation of team performance**, here are some indicators of **poor performance**:

- *Poor communication*: Communication is uneven. Team members don't listen to others or express opinions in a positive manner, and personality conflicts arise.
- *Poor problem solving*: Root cause analysis is not systematic or logical, so problems remain unresolved.
- *Lack of clarity*: Team members are unsure of their roles or responsibilities in the team or how the teamwork relates to strategic goals of the organization.
- **Inadequate management of timelines and *deadlines:*** Meetings are delayed or cancelled, projects are not completed on time, and reports are delayed.
- *Poor leadership*: The leader has no clear role and does not help the team to stay focused on tasks. Team members do not respect the leader
- *Lack of interest and skills*: Team members do not want to participate, have personal problems, or lack necessary training, skills, or expertise to complete tasks.

Patient Safety

Culture of Safety

DEVELOPING AN ORGANIZATION'S PATIENT SAFETY CULTURE

Developing an organization's **patient safety culture** reduces errors related to medications, treatment, patient care, and other adverse events. Assessment includes reviewing mortality rates, outcomes, best practices, critical pathways, accreditation reports, internal and external benchmarking, and comparative data. To develop a culture of patient safety, the CPHQ must:

- Identify the baseline.
- Establish an ongoing organizational vision directed at patient safety, with commitment by the governing board and upper management to allocation of financial, personnel, and time resources.
- Establish strategic plans to promote safety.
- Communicate organization-wide about the importance of safety, including education and training.
- Empower staff to identify errors and intervene to reduce risks.
- Identify systemic processes that provide opportunities for improving patient safety.

DEVELOPING AN ORGANIZATION'S PATIENT SAFETY CULTURE WITH AHRQ SURVEYS

Begin assessment of the organization's patient safety culture with a **survey**. The **Agency for Healthcare Research and Quality** (AHRQ) sponsors surveys for assessing patient safety in different healthcare organizations, including hospitals, nursing homes, and outpatient facilities.

Visit http://www.ahrq.gov/ for free downloads.

AHRQ's surveys are suitable for *all levels of staff* within the organization. The surveys ask questions related to safety, error in medications and treatments, and incident reporting. They typically take less than 15 minutes to complete, so these surveys could be completed as part of staff meetings or during clinical hours. The surveys use a scale of 1–5, checklists, and narrative responses. Sections include: Work area/unit; Supervisor/manager; Communications; Frequency of events reported; Patient safety goals; Hospital/Facility; Number of events reported; Background information; and Comments.

EFFECT OF EXTERNAL FORCES ON SAFETY CULTURE

The patient safety culture constantly evolves in response to new information, technology, and both internal and external forces. The **important external forces** that impact the development of an organization's patient safety culture are:

- *External regulations, legislation, and healthcare initiatives,* such as state and federal laws and Leapfrog, promote and mandate safe practices to improve patient safety and provide optimal, cost-effective care.
- *Accreditation agencies* provide mandates and standards for healthcare organizations and their leaders to reduce risk and improve patient safety. For example, the Joint Commission issued the National Practice Safety Guides (NPSG) to assist healthcare organizations in assessing and developing safe practices.

- ***Professional organizations***, such as the American Medical Association and the American Nurses association, have principles and codes of ethics that require quality care and patient safety.

EFFECT OF LEADERSHIP ON SAFETY CULTURE

Leadership is absolutely essential for developing the organization's patient safety culture because substantive change requires commitment from leadership to support the ideals of patient safety and provide the resources necessary to assess, train staff, and institute performance improvement methods to effect change. Leaders at all levels, from the governing board to the unit or department head, must work together to create a climate in which safety is expected as a first priority. Leadership must:

- ***Model safe practices***: Leaders must consistently consider and demonstrate safe practices as part of their functions.
- ***Preach safe practices***: Leaders must consistently address the need for safe practices and must provide information in support of patient safety.
- ***Facilitate safe practices***: Leaders must provide training, education, equipment, staff, and other resources necessary to establish a culture of safety within the organization

EFFECT OF MEDICAL ERRORS ON SAFETY CULTURE

Every assessment for patient safety culture must include a review of **medical errors,** which are unintentional but preventable mistakes in providing care. *Errors* are failures to carry out a planned action or using the wrong plan. *Adverse events* are the negative results of errors, such as injuries and deaths.

- Errors may result from ***commission*** (doing something) or ***omission*** (failing to do something).
- Errors can be ***active***, resulting from contact between the patient and an aspect of the medical system, such as a nurse or piece of equipment.
- Errors can be ***latent***, resulting from a failure of in system design.
- Error ***chains*** are the series of events that lead to a negative outcome, usually identified through root cause analysis.

Medical errors are most often identified after an adverse event occurs. Some go unidentified until they are found on medical record reviews. Typical errors include: Incorrect diagnoses; medications mistakes (such as wrong medication or dose); delays in reporting of results; communication failure; improper or inadequate care; and mistaken identity.

EFFECT OF DIVERSITY ISSUES ON SAFETY CULTURE

Account for **diversity** when establishing a patient safety culture. Differences related to ethnicity, religious, and cultural backgrounds might be easier to deal with than more institutionalized differences. Despite the best efforts of interdisciplinary teams and leadership, resistant subgroups of employees exist, such as those working in isolated areas, or those with a shared purpose or function, including such disparate groups as administrators, laboratory technicians, and housekeepers. Each group has its own perspective that must be respected. For example, within the organization there may be considerable differences in goals and perceptions between administrators and staff, and between doctors and nurses. Employees are often anxious regarding change and fear a loss of autonomy in working toward shared patient safety goals. Employees at all levels of the organization must be actively engaged in establishing a **patient safety culture**.

PATIENT SAFETY OFFICER

Effective patient safety programs need a full-time **patient safety officer**, trained and responsible for safety activities as their only occupation. The position should be one of high rank within the organization and invested with authority to make decisions and change processes to ensure safety. Responsibilities are to:

- Act as liaison officer for issues related to safety at all levels of the organization, and external agencies and organizations.
- Coordinate education and training activities and make safety presentations.
- Organize and coordinate with patient safety teams and other teams related to safety improvement.
- Provide periodic reviews and revisions of policies.
- Disseminate patient safety information and facilitate organization-wide communication.
- Establish a computerized error reporting system focused on process rather than individuals and punitive actions.
- Review medical error information, including trends and patterns.
- Establish rapid response teams and investigations processes.
- Complete risk assessment and risk management procedures.
- Facilitate performance measurement and staff incentive programs.

NCQA GUIDELINES

The National Committee for Quality Assurance (NCQA) addresses safety issues as part of its accreditation standards, in response to the Institute of Medicine's (IOM) call for accrediting agencies to ensure organizations focus on patient safety. Guidelines directed at managed care organizations provide useful information for all other organizations:

- Educate staff regarding clinical safety by providing information.
- Provide collaborative training within the network related to safe clinical practice.
- Combine data within the network [organization] on adverse outcomes/ polypharmacy.
- Make improving patient safety a priority for quality improvement activities.
- Provide and distribute information about safe practices that includes information about computerized pharmacy order systems, Intensive Care- trained physicians, best practices, research on safe clinical practices.

JOINT COMMISSION'S NATIONAL PATIENT SAFETY GOALS (2018)

Joint Commission issues **National Patient Safety Goals** annually for different healthcare programs; *hospital goals* are fairly representative:

- Improve accuracy of patient identification with two identifiers. Ensure right patient receives the right blood for transfusion.
- Improve timelines for reporting test results to the correct individual.
- Improve the safety of using medications with proper labeling, review of drugs with similar names or appearances, and reduction in anticoagulation therapy risks. Improve documentation and communication of patient medications.
- Improve medical alarm response by ensuring adequate volume.
- Reduce the risk of healthcare-associated infections by following WHO or CDC hand washing guidelines and treating healthcare-associated infections as sentinel events. Also, note special precautions for MDROs, central line-associated bloodstream infections, post-op, and UTIs from catheterization.

142

- Identify inherent patient safety risks, including the risk of suicide.
- Reduce errors in surgery by correctly identifying the patient receiving right surgery, marking the spot for incision, and taking a moment before operating to ensure everything is in order.

APPLYING THE JOINT COMMISSION'S SAFETY GOALS TO AN ORGANIZATION

The **Joint Commission (TJC)** issues the **National Patient Safety Goals** (NPSG), under advisement of national experts. Goals and implementation expectations are listed for various types of programs: Ambulatory care; assisted living; behavioral health care; critical-access hospital; disease-specific care; home care; hospital; laboratory; long-term care; networks; and office-based surgery.

First, identify those goals that apply to the organization. For example, the organization may have to comply with multiple safety standards related to hospitals, specific diseases, behavioral health, and laboratory programs. Each year the NPSG is updated. The organization must meet only those requirements that apply to the services it provides, and can bypass irrelevant requirements. The organization is responsible for compliance with NPSG requirements by staff, those granted privileges, and those with whom the organization has a contractual agreement.

JOINT COMMISSION INTERNATIONAL

The **Joint Commission International** (JCI) is a division of the Joint Commission Resources (JCR), the non-profit affiliate of the Joint Commission. The JCI provides **international accreditation** for safety and quality care for many types of healthcare organizations. The JCI provides an Internet-based software tool, the ***International Self-Assessment System*** (ISAS) to assist organizations to manage quality and to achieve compliance with standards. International organizations can benefit from accreditation because it provides evaluation and goals for improvement and establishes that the organization complies with international safety standards. JCI provides measurements for benchmarking and risk reduction strategies. Individuals and some insurance companies are looking at JCI-accredited international organizations that provide more cost-effective healthcare than the U.S.A. The JCI process is designed with country-specific accommodations related to laws, religion, and culture.

NATIONAL QUALITY FORUM

The **National Quality Forum** (NQF) is a non-profit membership organization for healthcare organizations interested in quality measurement and reporting to ensure better outcomes and patient safety. The goal of NQF is to promote national priorities for ***performance measurement*** and ***public reporting***, working in collaboration with other agencies and partners to reach consensus on a core set of measures. Membership is granted to organizations, rather than individuals, so the governing board and administration must determine if they want to participate at a national level in establishing guidelines. Member organizations can participate in the national dialogue and can participate in the forum through membership in one of the main member councils: Consumer, Purchaser, Health Professional, Provider and Health Plan, and Research and Quality Improvement. NQF provides valuable educational forums and publications for member organizations related to factors in quality improvement, such as reporting and consideration of environmental factors.

The **National Qualify Forum** (NQF) endorses a set of **safe practices** to assess and develop an organization's patient safety culture. According to NQF, the four elements needed to create and sustain a patient safety culture are:

- Leadership must ensure structures are in place for organization-wide awareness and compliance with safety measures, including adequate resources and direct accountability.
- Measurement, analysis, and feedback must track safety and allow for interventions.
- Team-based patient care with adequate training and performance improvement activities must be organization-wide.
- Safety risks must be continuously identified and interventions taken to reduce patient risk.

NQF SAFE PRACTICES

The **NQF Safe Practices** are:

1. Considering the rights and responsibilities of the patient; providing informed consent; respecting advance directives and patient's directions related to care; and providing full disclosure of medical error.
2. Providing adequate, well-trained and supervised staff and resources to meet healthcare needs, and Critical Care-certified physicians for ICU or CCU.
3. Managing information and care through proper documentation; providing prompt, accurate test results; utilizing standardized procedures for labeling diagnostic studies; and providing discharge planning.
4. Managing medications by implementing a computerized prescriber order entry (CPOE) system; standardizing abbreviations; maintaining updated medication lists for patients; including pharmacists in medication management and selecting a formulary; standardizing labeling; identifying high alert drugs; and dispensing drugs in unit doses.
5. Preventing healthcare-associated infections through ventilator bundle intervention; following best practices for central venous lines; complying with CDC hand washing guidelines; immunizing staff and patients for influenza; preventing surgical site infections through the appropriate use of antibiotics, proper hair removal, glucose control for cardiac patients, and temperature control for colorectal surgery.
6. Providing safe practices for surgery; informing patients of risks; taking measures to prevent errors such as operating on the wrong site; and using prophylactic treatments as indicated to prevent complications.
7. Providing procedures and ongoing assessment to prevent site-specific or treatment-specific adverse events, such as pressure ulcers, thromboembolism, deep vein thrombosis, allergic reactions, or anticoagulation complications.

INSTITUTE FOR HEALTHCARE IMPROVEMENT

The **Institute for Healthcare Improvement** (IHI) is a non-profit organization whose goal is to improve healthcare throughout the world. It provides both free and fee-based programs and services. IHI launched healthcare initiatives, and offers books, videos, and audiotapes to provide guidance in quality improvement. IHI produces a series of free white papers, such as *Leadership Guide to Patient Safety*, which outlines the eight steps an organization can follow to achieve patient safety. Much of the information provided by IHI is available free, including interactive tools for measuring adverse drug events and FMEA tools. IHI offers collaborative programs, such as the IMPACT Network, where organizations work together to facilitate changes at the system level, and Innovation Communities, which are collaborative learning laboratories. The patient safety guidelines cover broad areas and many apply to almost all healthcare organizations.

IHI 5 MILLION LIVES CAMPAIGN

The **Institute for Healthcare Improvement** (IHI) originally instituted a **100,000 lives campaign**, with over 3,000 hospitals participating over an 18-month period. The campaign was focused on implementing **six interventions** to avoid preventable loss of life:

- Deploy rapid response teams
- Deliver reliable, evidence-based care for acute MI
- Prevent adverse drug events
- Prevent central line infections
- Prevent surgical site infections
- Prevent ventilator-associated pneumonia

The **5 Million Lives Campaign** involved over 4,000 hospitals implementing **twelve interventions** this time over a 24-month period. The interventions included all six from the previous campaign while adding these six:

- Prevent harm from high alert medications
- Reduce surgical complications
- Prevent pressure ulcers
- Reduce methicillin-resistant *Staphylococcus aureus* (MRSA) infections
- Deliver reliable, evidence-based care for congestive heart failure to avoid readmissions
- Get boards on-board to accelerate organizational progress toward safe care

AHRQ QUALITY INDICATORS

The Agency for Healthcare Research and Quality (**AHRQ**) **Quality Indicators** are distributed as a software tool free of charge to healthcare organizations to help them to identify adverse events or potential adverse events that require further study. This software is invaluable in developing an organization's patient safety culture. Hospital discharges of patients over 18 years old are assessed for the following quality indicators:

- Complications of anesthesia; death in low mortality, diagnostic-related diseases (DRG); decubitus ulcer; failure to rescue; foreign body left in the patient during a procedure; iatrogenic pneumothorax; care-related infections.
- Post-operative hip fracture, hemorrhage or hematoma; physiologic or metabolic derangements; respiratory failure; pulmonary embolism, deep vein thrombosis, sepsis, or wound dehiscence in abdominopelvic surgeries.
- Accidental puncture, laceration, or transfusion reaction.
- Birth trauma.
- Obstetrical trauma from vaginal delivery with or without instruments or Caesarean section.

The data indicators may also be used to assess safety factors at an area (such as county) level per 100,000 population.

LEAPFROG

Leapfrog is a consortium of healthcare purchasers and employers that benefits millions of Americans. Leapfrog's initial focus was on reducing healthcare costs by preventing medical errors and "leaping forward" by rewarding hospitals and healthcare organizations that improve safety and quality of care. Leapfrog developed initiatives to improve safety, which can be valuable tools for assessing and developing a patient safety culture. Leapfrog provides an annual **Hospital and Quality Safety Survey** to assess progress. It releases regional data and encourages voluntary public reporting. Leapfrog instituted the Leapfrog Hospital Rewards Program (LHRP) as a pay-for-performance program to reward organizations for showing improvement in key measures.

LEAPFROG'S SAFE PRACTICES INITIATIVES

- Leapfrog's first initiative is ***preventing medical errors***. Purchasers of healthcare agree to base their purchases on four principals:
  - o Educating enrollees about patient safety and providing comparative performance data.
  - o Recognizing and rewarding healthcare organizations that demonstrate improvement in preventing errors.
  - o Making health plans accountable for implementing these principles.
  - o Advocating for these principles with clients by utilizing benefits consultants.
- Implementation of ***computerized physicians' order entry*** (CPOE) system that includes software to detect and prevent errors, with a goal of decreasing prescribing errors by more than 50%.
- ***Evidence-based hospital referral*** (EHR), requiring referral to hospitals that demonstrate the best results and experience related to high-risk conditions and surgeries, assessed according to the number of procedures/ treatments they do each year and outcomes data, with a goal of reducing mortality rates by 40%.
- ***ICU physician staffing*** requiring specially trained specialists (Intensivist) with a goal of reducing mortality rates by 40%.
- ***Leapfrog Safe Practices Score*** assesses the progress a healthcare organization is making on 30 safe practices that Leapfrog has identified as reducing the risk of harm to patients.

NATIONAL HEALTHCARE SAFETY NETWORK

The National Healthcare Safety Network (NHSN) integrates and replaces three separate programs: National Nosocomial Infections Surveillance (NNIS), Dialysis Surveillance Network (DSN), and National Surveillance System for Health Care Workers (NaSH). Participating in this program provides valuable ***comparative data***. All healthcare facilities, such as hospitals and dialysis centers, can participate in the Internet-based program that allows for reporting and sharing data. Those who apply to become members must agree to utilize CDC definitions, follow strict protocols, and submit data every six months. Anonymity of the institutions is protected. The program streamlines reporting of data and provides comparative data from across the United States. The system can identify sentinel or unusual events and notify appropriate participating agencies. There are three components to NHSN: Patient safety, healthcare worker safety, and research and development. Extensive data analysis features are part of the program. Reports of nosocomial, or hospital-acquired, infections that were previously issued by NNIS are now issued by NHSN.

Patient Safety Programs

DEVELOPING PATIENT SAFETY PROGRAMS

Each healthcare organization has unique needs and challenges to face in developing a patient safety program, although many components are universally needed. Facilitating development of a **patient safety program** requires planning and taking these steps:

- Identify a quality professional or interdisciplinary group to manage the safety program.
- Define the scope of the program, including risk identification, management, and response to adverse events.
- Provide mechanisms to integrate all aspects of the program into organization-wide functions.
- Establish procedures for rapid response to medical errors or adverse events.
- Establish procedures for both internal and external reporting of medical errors.
- Define and disseminate intervention strategies, such as risk reduction, risk tracking, and root cause analysis.
- Outline mechanisms for staff support related to involvement in sentinel events.
- Establish procedures and responsibilities for reporting to the governing board.

A **patient safety program** must include these components:

- Functional infrastructure with leader, safety officer, teams, and software for tracking and measures.
- Linkage of program goals with strategic goals of the organization.
- Establishment of policies and procedures to reduce and control risk, and supportive training.
- Reporting system to identify adverse events or incidents.
- Participation in national patient safety initiatives, such as NPSG, IPSG, IHI 5 Million Lives, and Leapfrog.
- Rapid response procedures to deal with medical errors and sentinel events.
- Adequate data collection procedures to ensure performance measurement, tracking, and data analysis.
- Performance improvement activities directed at specific goals.
- Documentation of all processes, procedures, reporting, and timelines.

PHYSICIAN PARTICIPATION IN A PATIENT SAFETY PROGRAM

Physician participation is a necessary component of any patient safety program. Physicians must be *active partners* in the organization's methods to reduce patient risk and improve risk management. Doctors, like other health professionals, are concerned that error reports are kept confidential and non-discoverable, and that evidence is used to improve processes, rather than for punitive actions. Involve physicians in the following:

- Identifying areas of potential risks in patient care processes.
- Designing risk reduction programs for clinical care.
- Developing criteria for identifying potential or actual clinical risk cases.
- Evaluating specific cases that have been identified as having risks.
- Actively participating in process improvement teams and risk management to promote patient safety and correct problems.

ENVIRONMENTAL STEPS IN A PATIENT SAFETY PROGRAM

Here are the steps to evaluate **environmental safety hazards and risks** for a safety program:

1. Prepare a written plan that clearly outlines environmental safety concerns, policies, and procedures.
2. Establish a safe environment for staff and patients, including fall prevention strategies, such as installing handrails, contrast strips on stairways, and analyzing work flow to facilitate functions.
3. Identify security risks, such as infant/child abduction, and establish processes to increase security, such as alarms, ID badges, locks, better lighting, and security officers.
4. Follow EPA and state regulations and educate staff about correct identification, handling, storage, and disposal of hazardous wastes, including corrosives, flammables, reactives, and toxics.
5. Conduct fire safety drills and check equipment and buildings for fire dangers.
6. Monitor medical equipment, ensuring routine maintenance, testing and regular inspection.
7. Evaluate power/utility requirements, including emergency power, and maintaining, testing, and inspecting utilities.
8. Designate individuals to monitor and coordinate environmental safety management and to develop procedures for dealing with threats/problems.
9. Complete a risk assessment of the physical plant, including buildings, grounds, equipment, and related systems, such as electrical, lighting, IT, ventilation, and plumbing.
10. Establish organization-wide safety policies and procedures, including no smoking policies.
11. Maintain the physical plant by monitoring and responding to product recalls.
12. Establish a plan for emergency preparedness; evaluate areas of vulnerability, test preparedness, response, and recovery times.
13. Establish an interdisciplinary team to identify opportunities for improvement and facilitate performance improvement processes.

> **Review Video: Fall Prevention**
> Visit mometrix.com/academy and enter code: 972452

INCORPORATING SYSTEMS AND INDIVIDUALS IN A PATIENT SAFETY PROGRAM

When developing a patient safety program, consider the errors that relate to **systems** and those that relate to **individuals** in the program design:

Systems: Most errors are related to inefficient or flawed systems, rather than individual error. Systems errors are the consequence of systemic deficiencies, such as inadequate staffing, insufficient third-party payments, poor maintenance, and outdated equipment, policies, and procedures. Some of these factors are internal, but others are external, so the organization has little control over them. Mitigate these factors as much as possible to improve safety.

Individuals: Humans make mistakes despite the best planning and systems, so plan ways to immediately identify and decrease errors, such as through computerized physician order entering (CPOE), bar coding, and triggers for data collection that allow for identification of errors so the effects are mitigated.

EVIDENCE-BASED PRACTICE

Use **evidence-based practice** (EBP) for integrating safety concepts into an organization. EBP is based on the best available scientific and clinical information, characterized as *"best practices."*

Although information about best practices is readily available, the best quality care is not always provided. Two examples of adverse events caused by ignoring EBP are:

- Failure to give Aspirin to a patient in the Emergency Room with a possible myocardial infarction, leading to blood clots.
- Treating a viral infection with antibiotics, which is inappropriate and of little value.

Utilizing EBP ensures that practitioners are aware of best practices and that systems are set up in such a way to influence their decision-making, such as through the use of:

- Clinical decision support system (CDSS).
- Computerized physician/provider order entry (CPOE).
- Establishing protocols and standing orders.

INTEGRATING QUALITY MANAGEMENT INTO PATIENT SAFETY CONCEPTS

Organizations that have already instituted a program of **quality management**, such as continuous quality improvement (CQI) or total quality management (TQM), are in a good position to integrate patient safety concepts within their organizations. The goal of quality management is to look at processes at all levels of an organization, identify opportunities for improvement, and institute change. Data collection, measurement, and analysis are already institutionalized, so the primary change is that the concept of **patient safety** must be identified as a high priority goal of quality management. Focus efforts on improving safety by using guides such as the National Patient Safety Goals (NPSG). Safety concepts are then automatically integrated through the assessment and performance improvement process.

SAFETY BY-LAWS, ADMINISTRATIVE POLICIES, AND PROCEDURES

Integrating patient safety findings into governance and management activities establishes the organization's commitment to patient safety. The by-laws should specify lines of authority and responsibility at all levels in the organization related to patient safety. The governing board establishes the method by which safety issues are reported, and this should include the designated person to report, a specific timeline, and reporting requirements. Patient safety responsibilities, based on patient safety findings, should be included in job descriptions and should be delineated as part of administrative policies and duties. Administrative policies must emphasize all departments and areas of the organization are required to participate in safety activities and respond to patient safety findings. Evaluate all existing procedures and processes organization-wide, revise them as necessary, and institute new procedures in response to findings.

DEVELOPING AND REVISING WRITTEN HOSPITAL SAFETY PLANS

The **hospital safety plan** is a major component in the quality improvement plan for the organization, which ensures safety concerns are integrated into assessment and action plans. However, the safety plan should focus directly on the organization's commitment to providing a safe environment. Include an **introductory section** that references the mission or vision statement of the organization, outlining how the safety plan relates to the strategic goals.

Next, explain the **scope** of the plan:

1. A **statement of purpose** that explains the main focus of the plan, such as "reduce mortality" or "improve patient care by identifying risks."
2. Specific **goals**, objectives, or priorities in performance improvement activities related to safety, with the steps to achieving these outlined.

3. Explanation of **responsibilities**, including those of the governing board, safety officer, staff members, patients, visitors, and volunteers.
4. Explain confidentiality.
5. Plan for evaluation.

Technology Resources

CLINICAL DECISION SUPPORT SYSTEM

Clinical decision support systems (CDSS) are interactive software applications that provide information to physicians or other healthcare providers to help with healthcare decisions. The programs contain a base of medical knowledge to which patient data can be entered, and an evidence-based inference system provides patient-specific advice. For example, a CDSS system may be used in the Emergency Department so that staff can enter symptoms into the program and, based on the information entered, the CDSS program provides possible diagnoses and treatment options. The CDSS system may be used for a variety of purposes:

- Record keeping and documentation, such as authorizations.
- Monitoring of patient's treatments, research protocols, orders, and referrals.
- Ensuring cost-effectiveness by monitoring orders to prevent duplication or tests that are not indicated by the condition, signs or symptoms.
- Providing support for physician diagnosis and ensuring treatments are based on best practices.

COMPUTERIZED PHYSICIAN/PROVIDER ORDER ENTRY SYSTEM

Computerized physician/provider order entry (CPOE) systems are clinical software applications that automate medication/treatment ordering, requiring that orders be typed in a standard format to avoid mistakes in ordering or interpreting orders. CPOE is promoted by Leapfrog as a means to reduce medication errors. About 50% of medication errors occur during ordering, so reducing this number can have a large impact on patient safety. Most CPOE systems contain a *clinical decision support system* (CDSS) too, so that the system can provide an immediate alert related to patient allergies, drug interactions, duplicate orders, or incorrect dosing at the time of data entry. Some systems can also provide suggestions for alternative medications, treatments, and diagnostic procedures. The CPOE system may be integrated into the information system of the organization for easier tracking of information and data collection. A CPOE system is cost-effective, replaces handwritten orders, and allows easy access to patient records.

BARCODE MEDICATION ADMINISTRATION

Barcode medication administration (BCMA) uses wireless mobile units at the point-of-care to scan the barcode on each unit of medication or blood component before it is dispensed. *Scanning* ensures the correct medication and dosage is given to the correct patient, eliminating most point-of-administration medication errors. The BCMA system can also be used for lab specimen collection, sorting, and testing. BCMA requires monitoring and input from Pharmacy, as each new barcode must be entered into the system. Additionally, some medications are received in bulk, so when they are dispensed in unit doses barcodes must be individually attached. Staff must be trained to ensure that BCMA is utilized properly and consistently. The FDA requires drug suppliers to provide barcodes on the labels of medications and biological products (e.g., vaccines). BCMA increases safety for patients, integrates with the medication administration record, and the information system of the organization, providing data for assessment of performance and performance improvement measures.

RADIO FREQUENCY IDENTIFICATION

Radio frequency identification (RFID) is an automatic tracking system that employs embedded digital memory chips, with unique codes, to follow patients, medical devices, medications, and staff. A chip can carry multiple types of data, such as expiration dates, patient's allergies, and blood types. A chip may be embedded in the identification bracelet of the patient and all medications for the patient tagged with the same chip. Chips have the ability to both read and write data, so they are more flexible than bar coding. The data on the chips can be read by sensors from a distance or through materials, such as clothes, although tags don't apply or read well on metal or in fluids. There are two types of RFID:

- **Active:** Continuous signals are transmitted between the chips and sensors.
- **Passive:** Signals are transmitted when in close proximity to a sensor.

Thus, a passive system may be adequate for administration of medications, but an active system would be needed to track movements of staff, equipment, or patients.

COMPUTERIZED NOTIFICATION SYSTEMS

The **computerized notification system** alerts physicians to **abnormal** laboratory or imaging results. Although this system ensures that alerts are communicated, some results are still lost, and physician follow-up is not always completed, especially in Ambulatory Care, where the physician may not see the patient on a regular basis. These steps improve safety and follow-up:

- Train physicians to check for computerized notices daily. Give clear explanations of the goals, needs, and responsibility for patient safety.
- Set the system to send an automatic notification to the sender when the receiver opens the alert message.
- Set the system to send an automatic second notification to the receiver if the alert message is not opened within a preset period of time.
- Set the system to send an automatic notification to the sender to contact the physician by other means if the second notification is not opened within a preset period of time.
- Monitor and evaluate physicians for compliance.

ELECTRONIC MEDICAL RECORDS

The **electronic medical record** (EMR) is a digital, computerized patient record, often integrated with CPOE and CDSS to improve patient care and reduce medical error. Software applications vary considerably and standardization has not yet been implemented, so the organization must carefully review its current and future anticipated needs against the compatibility of applications to interface with each other to provide for adequate measurements, data collection, reports, retrieval of data, analysis, and confidentiality. Physicians in private practice, especially those in large groups, often employ EMR, which may be different systems than those used in hospitals. Systems can be customized to meet the needs of the organization, but cost and lack of standardization remain barriers for implementation. However, there is a positive correlation between *comprehensive EMR systems* and *patient outcomes*. Quantifiable data about cost-effectiveness is difficult to calculate because savings are often in terms of saved time, fewer interventions, and reduced errors.

Patient Safety Issues

MEDICATION SAFETY

About 7,000 deaths yearly in the United States are attributed to **medication errors.** 1 in 5 doses of medication given to patients in hospitals is incorrect. Ensure patient safety with proper handling and administration of medications:

- Avoid error-prone abbreviations or symbols. The Joint Commission has established a list of abbreviations to avoid, but mistakes are frequent with other abbreviations, too. Avoid abbreviations and symbols altogether, or restrict them to a limited, approved list.

- Prevent errors from illegible handwriting. Enter orders into a computer program. Handwritten orders should be block printed to reduce errors.
- Institute bar coding and scanners that allow the patient's wristband and medication to be scanned for verification.
- Provide lists of similarly-named and look-alike medications to educate staff.
- Establish an institutional policy for administering of medications that includes protocols for verification of drug, dosage, time, and patient identification. Educate the patient about his or her medications.

SAFETY AND INFECTION CONTROL

Between 48,000 and 98,000 patients die each year in hospitals because of errors in patient safety. A caring environment must be a **safe environment** for patients and their families. Patient safety is impacted by these factors:

- **Staffing practices**: Patient-staff ratios are of primary importance, as fewer staff working longer hours results in more errors. This is especially true in critical care areas, such as NICU or PICU. The expertise of the staff is another important factor. An increased proportion of care (in hours) by registered nurses decreases both hospital stay and complications.
- **Infection control**: The rates of hospital infections have steadily increased because of antibiotic-resistant pathogens (such as *Staphylococcus aureus* and *MRSA*) that are now endemic in some institutions. Patients with invasive devices, such as central lines or ventilators, are at increased risk. Much infection is related to poor hand washing and infection control practices on the part of staff.

HAND DISINFECTION

CDC's HAND WASHING GUIDELINES

All patients are potentially infectious, so staff must wash their hands before and after every direct contact with a patient or when removing gloves. **Hand contamination** is one of the most common causes of person-to-person transmission of infection. Train all medical personnel in hand washing techniques and observe them regularly for compliance. Here is the **CDC's free procedure**, reprinted from http://www.cdc.gov/nceh/vsp/cruiselines/handwashing_guidelines.htm:

- Hands should be washed using soap and warm, running water.
- Hands should be rubbed vigorously during washing for at least 20 seconds with special attention paid to the backs of the hands, wrists, between the fingers and under the fingernails.
- Hands should be rinsed well while leaving the water running.
- With the water running, hands should be dried with a single-use towel.
- Turn off the water using a paper towel, covering washed hands to prevent re-contamination.

ALCOHOL-BASED RUBS

While soap and water hand washing has been the standard for many years, **alcohol-based rubs** used correctly, of adequate concentration, kill twice as much bacteria in the same amount of time. Alcohol rubs are less irritating to the hands than repeated washing. Staff must be trained in used and observed for compliance. Hand fires have occurred when staff members smoke with alcohol-wet hands. Sample procedure:

- *Hand disinfection* is done for at least 15 seconds by using an alcohol-based rub, such as Purell®, and should be done before and after contact with a patient or after removal of gloves.
- All hand surfaces should be thoroughly coated with the alcohol-rub, including between the fingers, the wrists, and under the nails, and then the hands rubbed together until the solution evaporates.
- Hands should not be rinsed.
- Alcohol-based rubs disinfect but do not mechanically clean hands, so hands that are dirty or contaminated should be washed first with soap and water.

PATIENT SAFETY GOALS REVIEW

The process of **patient safety goals review** is an important function to ensure that there is compliance with *safety standards*. A process may be chosen for review as part of regular monitoring or because outcomes show an opportunity for improvement. Determine the safety guidelines that will be used, for example, the Joint Commission's NPSG specific for hospitals. Perform interviews, observations, data collection and analysis. Identify and document how each safety guideline is implemented. For example, one safety guideline is to improve patient identification. Pose these questions to determine if this guideline is met:

- Does the patient wear an identification bracelet issued by Admitting?
- Does the provider check the bracelet?
- Does the provider ask for identifying information, such as birth dates?
- How consistently are these procedures followed?

Review Video: Patient Safety Goals
Visit mometrix.com/academy and enter code: 275502

Safety Principles

INNOVATIVE SYSTEMS THINKING

Innovative systems thinking and resource use among the healthcare team requires empowering staff to make decisions and to identify needs that require resource allocations. Administration must look for nursing leaders who are open to nontraditional methods and not afraid to change. Consider the **Star Model**, based on a star diagram, in which the points are: Strategy, Structure, Human Resources, Incentives, Information and Decision-making. Star has a core of systemic culture and values:

- Staff laziness or inability is rarely the root cause of systemic problems.
- There is more than one optimal system, depending on internal and external factors.
- One point is not more important than another.
- A change in one area usually necessitates a change in another.
- The culture and values cannot be changed directly, but only indirectly through action on one of the points.
- Ingrained cultures and values can impede progress.

STEPS TO SYSTEMS THINKING

System thinking is a critical thinking approach to problem solving that takes an organization-wide perspective. Introduce systems thinking when there is lack of consensus, effective change is stalemated, and standards are inconsistent. Follow these steps:

- ***Define the issue***: Describe the problem in detail. Do not judge or offer solutions.
- ***Describe behavior patterns***: List factors related to the problem. Use graphs to outline possible trends.
- ***Establish cause-effect relationships***: Use the Five Whys or another root cause analysis method, or feedback loops.
- ***Define patterns of performance/behavior***: Determine how variables affect outcomes and the types of patterns of behavior currently taking place.
- ***Find solutions***: Discuss possible solutions and outcomes.
- ***Institute performance improvement activities***: Make process changes and then monitor for changes in behavior.

PROMOTING ORGANIZATIONAL VALUES AND COMMITMENT

System thinking focuses on how systems ***interrelate***, with each part affecting the entire system. For the CPHQ to promote organizational values and commitment, the organization must embrace systems thinking and its associated concepts:

- ***Individual responsibility***: Encourage individual workers to establish their own goals within the organization and to work toward a purpose.
- ***Learning process***: Respect the internalized beliefs of the staff and build upon these beliefs to establish a mindset based on continuous learning and improvement.
- ***Vision***: Share the organizational vision to help staff understand the purpose of change and to build commitment.
- ***Team process***: Assist teams to develop good listening and collaborative skills, so dialog increases and they are able to reach consensus.
- ***Systems thinking***: Encourage staff members to understand the interrelationship of all members of the organization and to appreciate how any change affects the whole.

155

CONSIDERING PATIENT CHARACTERISTICS

The synergy method for patient care recognizes that there are a number of **patient characteristics** that must be considered when matching a staff member's competencies to the needs of the patient and his or her family:

- **Resiliency** is the ability to recover from a devastating illness and regain a sense of stability, both physically and emotionally. Things that support resiliency are faith, a positive sense of hope, and a supportive network of friends and family.
- **Vulnerability** means the patient is susceptible to infection; has increased risk for disease; recovery is slowed; or is non-compliant because of anxiety, fear, lack of support, chronic illness, prejudice, and lack of information.
- **Stability** allows a patient and family to maintain a state of physical and/or emotional equilibrium despite illness and challenges. Important factors include: Relief from stress, conflicts, or emotional burdens; motivation; and values.
- **Complexity** occurs when more than one system is involved, and these can be internal (cardiac and renal systems) or external (addicted and homeless) or some combination (ill with poor family dynamics).

HUMAN FACTOR ENGINEERING

Human factor engineering is the discipline involved in trying to identify those things related to engineering and manufacturing and human interaction that may lead to errors, such as two different medications that look alike or different manufacturers for the same type of equipment. Human factor engineering includes assessing tasks involved in processes, including the physical, skill, and knowledge requirements, as well as the environment (heat, light, distractions) and equipment design. A number of different approaches are utilized to address safety:

- **Testing usability:** Identifying "workarounds" that staff members develop to cope with poor design or practice in order to improve efficiency or save time but can lead to serious errors.
- **Forcing function:** Taking action that prevents an error or requiring a specific step before another can be performed.
- **Utilizing standardization:** Using checklists and standardized equipment and processes to prevent errors.
- **Evaluating resiliency:** Considering how the organization anticipates change/problems and handles them.

HIGH-RELIABILITY ORGANIZATIONS

High-reliability organizations are those that involve hazardous work or environment but lower than usual occurrence of adverse events. All healthcare organizations strive for high-reliability but errors and adverse events remain common. Principles of high-reliability organizations include:

- **Constant concern regarding failure:** The organization recognizes risks inherent in healthcare and is constantly on the alert for areas/situations that may produce errors and makes use of human factor engineering.
- **Focus on promoting resilience:** The organization responds quickly to problems/errors and has the ability to identify threats before they cause harm.
- **Attention to operations:** Healthcare workers report problems and unsafe conditions when they observe them and are provided some autonomy in dealing with problems and unsafe conditions.

- **Adequate communication:** Documentation standards are adhered to and handoff procedures are standardized.
- **Promotion of culture of safety:** Safety is a concern at all levels in the organization and staff members are rewarded rather than intimidated for reporting safety concerns.

Risk Management

RISK MANAGEMENT PROCESS

Risk management is an organized, formal method of decreasing liability, financial loss, and risk or harm to patients, staff, or others by assessment and strategies. Risk management is driven by the insurance industry to minimize costs, and by quality managers to ensure quality healthcare and process improvement. A risk management program usually has a manager and specially trained staff responsible for:

- **Risk identification**, which begins with an assessment of current processes to identify and prioritize those that require further study to determine risk exposure.
- **Risk analysis**, which requires careful documenting of process through flow charts and root cause analysis, with each step in the process assessed for potential risks.
- **Risk prevention**, which involves identifying and training responsible teams to institute corrective or preventive processes.
- **Assessment and evaluation** of corrective and preventive processes is ongoing, to determine if they are effective or require modification.

EARLY WARNING SYSTEM

Risk management is concerned with decreasing liability and increasing safety. Integrating the outcomes of risk management assessment into the performance improvement process requires an organization-wide commitment to **reducing risk**. The governing board and CPHQ ensure that risk management assessments are considered when formulating mission and vision statements and strategic goals. Risk management assessment is one of the first concerns during process evaluation and process improvement. An **organization-wide early warning system** should be in place to screen patients for potential risks and identify:

- **Adverse patient occurrences (APO)**, unexpected events that negatively impact the patient's health or welfare.
- **Potentially compensable events (PCE),** which are APO's that may result in claims against the organization because of their negative impact on the patient's health or welfare.

If the organization has set up a method to quickly identify problems, then risks are minimized.

DEVELOPING OR REVISING WRITTEN PLANS FOR RISK MANAGEMENT PROGRAM

The **written risk management plan**, while not required by accreditation agencies, is usually required by liability insurers. The written plan must include:

- **Statement of purpose**: Outline the organization's general policy of risk management, such as patient safety guidelines or financial risk reductions.
- **Goals**: Make goals specific and measurable.
- **Program scope**: Include linkages with other programs.
- **Lines of authority**: Begin with the governing board and end with employees. Outline the responsibilities at each level.
- **Policies**: Include confidentiality (HIPAA) and conflict of interest policies.
- **Data sources and referrals**: Outline the types of measures the organization uses.
- **Documentation/reporting**: Clarify who is responsible for reporting. List the frequency of reports.

ACTIVITIES INTEGRATION

- *Evaluation of program*: Method and frequency of evaluation.
- *Charts and Diagrams*: Attach flow charts, organizational charts, and pertinent diagrams to the written risk management plan.

EMERGENCY MEDICAL TREATMENT AND ACTIVE LABOR ACT

The Emergency Medical Treatment and Active Labor Act (EMTALA) prevents patient "dumping" from emergency departments (ED) and concerns risk management, requiring staff training for compliance:

- Transfers from ED may be intrahospital or to another facility.
- Stabilization of the patient with emergency conditions or active labor must be done in the ED prior to transfer.
- Patient screening must be given prior to inquiring about insurance or the ability to pay.
- Stabilization requires treatment for emergency conditions and the doctor must have a reasonable belief that, although the emergency condition may not be completely resolved, the patient's condition will not deteriorate during transfer.
- Women in the ED in active labor should deliver both the child and placenta before transfer.
- The receiving department or facility should be capable of treating the patient and dealing with possible complications.
- Transfer to another facility is indicated if the patient requires specialized services not available intrahospital, such as to a burn center or NICU.

PROFESSIONAL LIABILITY

Risk manager must define **professional liability** for staff and ensure that related risks are minimized. Direct care providers must obtain written consents for Medicare, provide adequate care, and obey drug laws.

- *Physicians are liable for*: Misdiagnoses; lack of staff supervision; providing incorrect or substandard treatment; treating patients outside their area of expertise; failing to provide follow-up care; failing to seek necessary consultation; infections resulting from procedures; premature discharge; and lack of proper documentation.
- *Nurses are liable* **for**: Improper administration of drugs; failing to follow standard medical procedures; failing to follow physicians' written orders; taking incorrect verbal orders; failing to report changes in patients' conditions or defective equipment; miscounting sponges; instruments; and surgical equipment; avoidable injuries to patients from falls or burns; and mishandling patients' personal belongings.

NEGLIGENCE

Risk managers must determine the burden of proof for acts of **negligence**, including compliance with duty, breaches in procedures, degree of harm, and cause. Negligence means *proper care* was not provided, based on established standards. *Reasonable care* uses rationales for decision-making in relation to providing care. State regulations regarding negligence vary, but all have some statutes of limitation. The types of negligence are:

- *Negligent conduct,* which indicates that an individual failed to provide reasonable care or failed to protect or assist another, based on standards and their level of expertise.
- *Gross negligence* is willfully providing inadequate care, while disregarding the safety and security of another.

- *Contributory negligence* involves the injured party contributing to his or her own harm (e.g., a drug addict who overdoses).
- *Comparative negligence* determines the percentage amount of negligence attributed to each individual involved.

LOSS AND RISK EXPOSURE

Risk management includes *loss prevention*, taking proactive measures to eliminate loss, and *loss reduction*, taking reactive measures to decrease potential loss. Risk managers must identify risk exposure through continuous data collection of occurrences or adverse events, including external review, patient complaints, financial audits, referrals, observations, contracts, current litigation, and risky practices. Continuous analysis must also be conducted in these areas:

- *Liability*, including malpractice and defamation actions;
- *Employer-related issues*, including Workers Compensation, hiring, terminating, intellectual property losses, and death or disability of employees.
- *Property and environment issues*, including injuries related to equipment or Physical Plant, chemical or nuclear wastes, and transportation vehicles,
- *Financial or contract issues*, including embezzlement, theft, anti-trust actions related to peer review, contracts, fraud and abuse, and securities violations.

RISK AVOIDANCE AND PREVENTION

Risk management aligns with quality management in determining measures for **risk avoidance** and prevention. In the analysis process, adverse events may be shown to relate to dysfunction in the organization, increasing risk exposure, so risk managers must take steps to decrease this exposure:

- *Financial management* includes determining both risk retention and risk transfer:
- *Risk retention* occurs when the organization assumes financial responsibility for risks.
- *Risk transfer* occurs when financial responsibility for risks is transferred to an insurance company through policies.
- *Risk event control* involves development of specific programs and processes to limit risk exposure:
- *Avoidance* eliminates that which causes risk, such as a particularly high-risk neonatal program.
- *Shifting* changes internal responsibility for risk to external through contract services or referrals.
- *Prevention* changes processes to reduce adverse events, such as using disposable equipment to reduce infection rates.

CLAIMS MANAGEMENT

Risk management involves administrative functions like **claims management** and taking action on potentially compensable events (PCE), those liability events that may incur costs to the organization. The steps for claims management are:

- *Plan ahead:* The organization must be prepared with a plan to deal with different types of PCE, such as disability claims.
- *Evaluation:* A complete examination of the incident/claim should be undertaken as soon as possible to gather information, to determine liability, and decide whether it would be cost-effective to offer a settlement.

160

- ***Document carefully***: Proper documentation must be a continuous, proactive process, rather than reactive.
- ***Consult with insurance companies/Workman's Compensation and legal experts:*** Provide information to assist insurers to make decisions about claims and retain legal assistance as needed.
- ***Provide support and assistance***: Being responsive to the needs of claimants may avoid a liability suit.
- ***Maintain financial records***: Carefully maintain records of claims management costs.

MORTALITY REVIEWS

The risk of dying in a healthcare institution varies widely from one facility to another, with mortality rates twice as high in some institutions as in others; thus, **mortality reviews** are a critical element of risk management. Mortality reviews are conducted to determine if treatments and patient care were adequate and appropriate, and if any deaths were preventable, with the goal of reducing mortality. Mortality review includes ***mortality data*** and ***individual case review***. When establishing a procedure for mortality review, select a timeframe or number of consecutive deaths, and investigate all deaths that occurred during the timeframe or consecutively to the established number. Mortality review steps are:

- Screen for deaths, manually or electronically.
- A non-physician team performs an initial analysis to determine if further evaluation is needed, or if each case was unavoidable.
- Physicians review the avoidable cases for medical management, and a multidisciplinary team reviews them for patient care processes.
- A final peer review is conducted by physicians, departments and management for process and root cause analyses.

ROLE IN QUALITY MANAGEMENT

The **mortality review** is an important tool for quality management because it presents quantifiable information that provides opportunities for improvement. Mortality reviews include not only the total death rates of the organization, but by department, and are compared with external data. When reviewing mortality rates and targeting areas for improvement, consider the number of:

- Patients who were poor surgical risks.
- Deaths in the Emergency Department.
- Patients with "do not resuscitate" (DNR) orders.
- Patients who were terminal on admission.
- Patients whose hospital stays were lengthened, rather than transferring them to extended care facilities.
- Deaths attributed to hospital-acquired and community-acquired infections.
- Patterns of death by department or physician that suggest poor quality care or negligence.
- Patients referred for peer review before and after the mortality review.
- In-service education and training sessions.

MORTALITY REVIEW AND MEASUREMENT OF OUTCOMES

Mortality review is an efficient **measure of outcomes**. When faced with the need for performance improvement organization-wide, quality professionals may have an enormous number of improvement opportunities, all requiring assessment, prioritizing, and plans, which is time-consuming and causes delays in improving processes, so mortality rates are a good beginning point for these reasons:

- Deaths must be recorded and reported with cause of death, so data is readily available and easy to access.
- Deaths provide quantifiable data.
- Mortality rates are good indicators of overall quality performance.
- The mortality review helps to identify patterns and areas of concern within the organization.
- Because mortality reviews are retrospective, the search for information and records is simplified.
- Understanding the reason for mortality rates helps to establish performance improvement activities that directly target causes.

INTEGRATION OF RISK MANAGEMENT WITH QUALITY MANAGEMENT

Risk management must integrate with quality management as part of process improvement. Risk management holds a central role in quality management because it focuses on achieving positive outcomes and reducing risks and liability. Both quality management and risk management share the commitment to providing optimal care and utilizing measurement and data regarding incidents, performance surveillance, root cause analysis, and feedback to evaluate, design, and monitor processes. *Risk managers* must be familiar with accreditation and state regulatory statutes in relation to both risk management and quality management. State regulations vary in regard to confidentiality and immunity, and in some states, documentation related to quality measures and risk concerns must be maintained separately. However, the Joint Commission's standards require that quality management and risk management be linked.

ACTIVITIES IMPROVING PATIENT SAFETY

Patient safety performance improvement activities are campaigns to reduce error or improve patient outcomes. For example, a campaign to reduce postoperative infections involves performance improvement activities for surgeons, O.R. staff, ward staff, housekeeping staff, Environmental Services, Infection Control, Microbiology, patients' families, and allied health workers. The scope could be limited to one type of patient — diabetic kidney/pancreas transplant patients, for example — or could be broader, involving all surgical patients for June–December. A multidisciplinary problem like this one may involve: Surveillance; new Purchasing contracts; new vaccinations; translations; training; rescheduling workflow and worksites; and procedure modifications (e.g., monitoring air flow to negative-pressure rooms and placing hand antiseptics in every room). Performance and process improvement are central to the Joint Commission's *accreditation standards*. Begin by reading the standards to flag possible improvement activities. Next, look at the collected data that pertains to those flags. Teams must decide what to measure, how to collect data, brainstorm solutions, and then implement solutions in a concerted effort.

INTEGRATING THE JOINT COMMISSION'S PATIENT SAFETY GOALS INTO ORGANIZATIONAL ACTIVITIES

The **Joint Commission (TJC),** under advisement of national experts, issues the **National Patient Safety Goals** (NPSG), and the organization must ensure that the safety goals are integrated into organizational activities. TJC requires that organizations be in continuous compliance, but the organization may file to use a different approach or indicate the types of measurements being used. Leadership must establish high priority for compliance with safety goals and ensure that the organization is at 90% compliance throughout the 12-month period before resurvey. This may require redefining patient care and development of new processes. Those who are *noncompliant* receive an RFI (requirement for improvement), which is used as part of the accreditation survey, so internal measurement and assessment must be conducted. Compliance with NPSG requirements is made public. New requirements may have a phase-in period, with testing at 3, 6, and 9 months, and implementation rules must be followed carefully.

INTEGRATING JCI'S INTERNATIONAL PATIENT SAFETY GOALS INTO ORGANIZATIONAL ACTIVITIES

International healthcare organizations vary widely in their quality of care and attention to patient safety, depending on resources, training, national regulations, and standards. However, organizations accredited by the **Joint Commission International** can begin by focusing on integrating the **International Patient Safety Goals** through intensive staff education programs and monitoring for compliance:

- *Identify patients correctly*: Use *two* identifiers for medicines, blood, or blood products.
- *Checklist before beginning surgery*: Confirm the correct patient, procedure, and body part.
- *Improve effective communication*: Establish a process for taking orders and reports. Read back verbal and telephone orders.
- *Remove concentrated electrolytes* from patient care units, including potassium.
- *Surgical checklist*: Ensure proper documentation and the necessary equipment is in working order.
- *Mark surgical sites* with clear, identifiable markings.
- Comply with hand washing standards according to the CDC guidelines.
- *Assess risk of falls* and eliminate risks.

INTEGRATING NQF PATIENT SAFETY GOALS INTO ORGANIZATIONAL ACTIVITIES

The **National Quality Forum** (NQF) is a non-profit membership organization for healthcare organizations interested in furthering patient safety through quality measurement and reporting to ensure better outcomes, aiming to set standards for measurement of healthcare performance. Organizations engaged in process improvement must develop adequate processes for measurement and analysis, and the NQF can help to provide information and analysis. One of the goals of NQF is that standards of measurement be *NQF-endorsed*, so work with NQF guidelines and take advantage of outreach programs and educational offerings when establishing and integrating new processes for measurement. It facilitates the use of comparative data. NQF published national priorities and goals in April 2008, followed by activities to assist organizations with development of their action plans. While many of the objectives of NQF are not yet realized, integrating currently existing best practices can facilitate full implementation later.

INTEGRATING IHI PATIENT SAFETY GOALS INTO ORGANIZATIONAL ACTIVITIES

The **Institute for Healthcare Improvement** (IHI) is a non-profit organization whose goal is to improve healthcare throughout the world. Information from IHI related to patient safety goals can be easily integrated into organizational activities. Members can participate in conferences, seminars, and Internet-based programs. Materials can be utilized for training purposes as guidelines are based on best practices that readily apply to healthcare organizations. *Materials* that are available include:

- Guides to improvement in specific areas, such as decreasing ventilator-associated infections.
- Evidence-based processes for change.
- Tools, such as protocols, forms, and guidelines.

- Links to Internet resources.
- Literature reviews.

Because much of the information is free and downloadable from the IHI website, material specific to the needs of the organization can be included in education and training and used for integration of safety goals. Visit http://www.ihi.org/ihi for details.

INCIDENT REPORT REVIEW

Incident report review is part of risk management because incidents represent a failure in the system. Incident reports may be filled out by individuals who are involved in the incident, or who observed the incident. Increasingly, incident reports are generated by electronic data that indicates an error occurred, such as in medication administration. Incident report reviews are less comprehensive and time-consuming and more cost-effective than retrospective medical record reviews but can yield valuable information. Provide staff with incentives for reporting and assure them that confidentiality will be maintained. Incidents are grossly underreported in healthcare organizations. Reviews help determine if incidents are being accurately reported, so patterns and trends are identified early. The CPHQ may interview physicians and staff. A review looks at the incident in terms of process steps and determines where in the process an error occurred in order to establish a plan for improvement.

SENTINEL EVENT REVIEWS

Sentinel events are unexpected occurrences that result in *death, significant morbidity, or the risk of either*. These are "special cause" variations in the data, outside of normal variations, and must trigger further analysis if the event either happened within an organization or is related to services provided by an organization. Review includes:

- Utilization of established process for review of sentinel events.
- Completion of root cause analysis, which must include participation of leadership and all those involved in the process, and a review of standard practices and literature.
- Action plan formulated to reduce the risk of recurrence of the adverse event, indicating those responsible for implementing and monitoring the action plan.
- Time lines for compliance with action plans and outcomes.
- Training provided as necessary.
- Action plan piloted, modified as needed, implemented, and reviewed.
- Documentation of the complete sentinel event review process.

ROOT CAUSE ANALYSIS

Root cause analysis (RCA) is a retrospective attempt to determine the cause of a *sentinel event*, such as an unexpected death, or a cluster of events. Root cause analysis involves interviews, observations, and reviews of medical records. Often, an extensive questionnaire is completed by the professional doing the RCA, tracing essentially every step in the patient's hospitalization and care, including each treatment, each medication, and each contact. RCA focuses on systems and processes, rather than blaming individuals. How did the system break down? Where did the problem arise? In some cases, there may be one root cause, but in others, the causes may be multiple. The RCA must include a thorough literature review to ensure that process improvement plans based on the results of the RCA reflect current best practices. Plans without RCA are non-productive. If, for example, an infection is caused by contaminated air, process improvement plans to increase disinfection of the Operating Room surfaces would be ineffective.

FAILURE MODE AND EFFECTS ANALYSIS (FMEA)

Failure mode and effects analysis (FMEA) is a team-based prospective analysis method that attempts to identify and correct failures in a process **before utilization** to ensure positive outcomes. The steps for FMEA are:

1. ***Definition***: Describe the entire process and outline the scope of the FMEA.
2. ***Team creation***: Assemble a temporary, interdisciplinary *ad hoc* team for a specific FMEA process, whose members are involved in the process or have necessary expertise.
3. ***Description***: Create a flow chart, number each step in the process consecutively, and letter each sub-step consecutively. Complex processes require focus and prioritizing. Generate a final, permanent document with all the steps.
4. ***Brainstorming***: Discuss each step and sub-step for potential failure modes, considering major categories such as people, processes, equipment, and environment. Make an affinity diagram. Number and letter possible failures to correspond with the steps and sub-steps on the flow chart.
5. **Identify potential causes of potential failures:** Create a cause and effect diagram. Conduct root cause analysis or utilize Five Whys, and record potential causes on a worksheet.
6. **List potential adverse outcomes:** Identify the results of failures to the patient.
7. **Assign a severity rating:** Rate each potential adverse outcome (identified in step 6) on a scale of 1–10 for severity of the failure, with 1 being a slight annoyance and 10 being death.
8. **Assign an occurrence rating:** Rate each potential failure on a scale of 1–10, with 1 (remote) being a frequency of 1:10,000 and 10 (very high), being a frequency of 1:20, showing the probability of the failure occurring within a specified time period, usually a year.
9. **Assign a detection rating:** Rate each potential failure on a scale of 1–10 to determine the likelihood that hazards, errors, or failures will be identified prior to their occurrence. 1 (very high) is a 9/10 probability errors will be detected. 10 (remote) is a 0/10 probability errors will be detected.
10. **Calculate the Risk Priority Number (RPN):** Calculate the criticality index with this formula:
    a. Take the results of all three scales from steps 7, 8 and 9, i.e., **S**everity, **O**ccurrence, and **D**etection
    b. Multiply (S × O × D) to find the RPN
11. **Reduce potential failures:** The team brainstorms control measures to reduce or eliminate potential failures and identifies where in the process to place control measures. A leader is assigned to monitor and pilot test the control measures.
12. **Identify performance measures:** Introduce measures to monitor the modified process and reduce the RPN.

Practice Test #1

1. According to the Institute of Medicine, which of the following is NOT one of the domains of quality care?

    a. Government regulation.
    b. Customization.
    c. Safety.
    d. Interventions consistent with the latest medical findings.

2. Which of the following groups is least likely to report errors?

    a. Primary care physicians.
    b. Support staff.
    c. Independent contractors.
    d. Nurses.

3. Which of the following is NOT one of the types of quality problems identified by the Institute of Medicine's National Roundtable on Health Care Quality?

    a. Misuse.
    b. Abuse.
    c. Overuse.
    d. Underuse.

4. In behavioral health, the most important sentinel event for root cause analysis is:

    a. discharge.
    b. death.
    c. recovery.
    d. medication error.

5. It is easy to conduct a survey of medication-related errors because:

    a. there are very few of them relative to other types of error.
    b. deaths caused by such errors are rarely discovered.
    c. such errors have small but noticeable effects on health care costs.
    d. prescription-drug use is common and well documented.

6. In a successful lean healthcare facility, the largest costs related to quality will be incurred by:

    a. preventive efforts.
    b. internal failures.
    c. assessment programs.
    d. external failures.

7. When is the best time to discuss the results of a meeting exit survey?

    a. Immediately upon receiving the responses.
    b. At the beginning of the next meeting.
    c. Via email in the interim before the next meeting.
    d. These results should not be discussed.

8. Whenever possible, medication orders should be by:

a. weight.
b. volume.
c. dose.
d. strength.

9. What is the best explanation for the relatively slow introduction of lean practices into medical laboratories?

a. The variability and complexity of the samples in a laboratory are much higher than in a manufacturing environment.
b. Scientists are less receptive to the core principles of lean.
c. Medical laboratories function differently than factories.
d. Medical research is mostly funded by the government.

10. A simple but effective way for managers to obtain the support of team members is to:

a. threaten punishment.
b. ask for it.
c. mandate it.
d. ignore the team members.

11. A delay in discharging patients is likely to cause recurrent bottlenecks in:

a. admissions from the emergency room.
b. the filling of prescriptions.
c. admissions from surgical wards.
d. all of the above.

12. Which of the following conditions should a quality assessment program NOT examine?

a. A condition that is thought to be treatable.
b. A condition for which the treatment is susceptible to significant influence by health care providers.
c. A condition that has cost-effective treatments.
d. A rare condition that has a small effect on mortality or morbidity.

13. A doctor fails to administer an indicated test, and the patient's condition deteriorates to the point that he must be admitted to an inpatient facility. This is an example of:

a. preventive error.
b. treatment error.
c. diagnostic error.
d. communication error.

14. When is the best time for chairing during a meeting?

a. One hour beforehand.
b. At the beginning.
c. In the middle.
d. At the end.

15. Which of the following does NOT contribute to evidence-based practice in healthcare?

a. Clinical expertise.
b. Evidence collected by expert panels.
c. Tradition.
d. Patient preferences.

16. Which of the following is vastly different from the others?

a. SIPOC.
b. DMAIC.
c. PDCA.
d. PDSA.

17. In the perfect lean enterprise, delivery to the customer is:

a. instantaneous.
b. rapid.
c. customizable.
d. optional.

18. A presentation on the basic structures and processes of clinical governance would be most useful:

a. for small teams of employees.
b. for the organization as a whole.
c. for the directorate.
d. for individual employees.

19. A hospital-wide set of professional standards is important because it:

a. reduces the waste of time and resources.
b. eliminates bottlenecks.
c. encourages duplication.
d. minimizes the need for communication.

20. What is one disadvantage of the visioning strategy for setting goals?

a. It isolates team members.
b. It tends to bring internal conflicts to the surface.
c. The group must have at least six members for it to be feasible.
d. It tends to reinforce group norms.

21. Before conducting a safety audit in an emergency department, an administrator must first obtain:

a. a list of the employees in that department.
b. a map of the department.
c. a written set of safety standards.
d. statistics on adverse events.

22. During a meeting, the facilitator notices that one of the participants is getting agitated. After the meeting, what would be the best question for the facilitator to ask the participant?

    a. "Why are you so angry?"
    b. "What didn't you like about the meeting?"
    c. "Were you feeling irritated during the meeting?"
    d. "Don't you hate it when your coworkers act that way?"

23. The process chain in a laboratory is particularly subject to:

    a. variability.
    b. delay.
    c. disorganization.
    d. conflict.

24. Research suggests that the largest proportion of adverse events attributable to negligence occur in the:

    a. post-trauma unit.
    b. surgery unit.
    c. maternity ward.
    d. emergency room.

25. Which of the following is the source of the most medication errors?

    a. Orders that require lab results.
    b. High-risk orders.
    c. Automatic orders.
    d. Verbal orders.

26. Which of the following is NOT one of the typical questions in a force-field analysis?

    a. "What do you hope to accomplish in the meeting?"
    b. "What was bad about the meeting?"
    c. "What was good about the meeting?"
    d. "How can we improve meetings in the future?"

27. The definitive proof of the success of a regulation program is:

    a. fewer complaints from customers.
    b. a decreased need for inspections.
    c. a boost in employee morale.
    d. an increase in throughput.

28. A hospital manager notices that a significant proportion of medication errors in the facility involve the same two drugs. What is the most likely cause of this?

    a. The drugs are widely available.
    b. The drugs are made by the same company.
    c. The drugs come in similar packaging.
    d. The drugs are habit-forming.

29. One advantage of the kaizen approach to DMAIC implementation is that:

    a. it replicates the project-team approach.
    b. all of the team members are involved in all phases of the process.
    c. it can be performed while employees complete their normal tasks.
    d. it is accomplished in about a week.

30. The practice of waiting for a certain number of samples before commencing a test run results in:

    a. fewer bottlenecks.
    b. more bottlenecks.
    c. shorter lead times.
    d. longer lead times.

31. A whole systems approach to clinical governance is important because:

    a. it isolates particular areas of concern.
    b. it can be administered within one week.
    c. changes must be applied at all levels of the organization.
    d. delays in service provision are rare.

32. Because of a doctor's poor handwriting, a prescription must be reworked before it leaves the pharmacy. Which of the following is true?

    a. The doctor should be reprimanded.
    b. The pharmacy should incorporate bar coding.
    c. The prescription should not count towards the pharmacy's yield.
    d. The error should be reported to the FDA.

33. A hospital manager finds that he is unable to effectively supervise all of the employees who report directly to him. A reorganization of the hospital hierarchy should:

    a. eliminate some of the subordinate employees.
    b. reallocate material resources.
    c. minimize the manager's span of control.
    d. call for the hiring of another manager.

34. Hospitals that implement computerized provider order entry (CPOE) almost always see a decline in:

    a. medication errors.
    b. diagnostic errors.
    c. adverse events.
    d. latent errors.

35. In a traditional meeting, the timekeeper and the minute-taker roles are:

    a. filled by different people every time.
    b. filled by the same person.
    c. filled by the same two people in each meeting.
    d. filled by employees who are not required to participate in the meeting.

36. An adverse drug reaction can be best described as:

a. an unforeseen side effect of the administration of a drug.
b. the interaction of one drug with another drug being administered at the same time.
c. harm that occurs during or after the administration of a drug.
d. harm that occurs as a result of the administration of a drug.

37. A meeting of department managers is discussing the catering service and menu for a hospital-wide special occasion. This decision should be made by:

a. building a consensus.
b. voting.
c. fiat.
d. brainstorming.

38. Confronted by excessive WIP levels, many laboratories take the unhelpful step of:

a. decreasing the number of test runs.
b. acquiring a larger laboratory.
c. hiring more employees.
d. installing new technology.

39. When establishing a clinical-governance training program for the directorate, it is useful to:

a. align the subject matter with the specific tasks of the audience.
b. eschew case studies.
c. emphasize the basic concepts of clinical governance.
d. customize instruction for each person.

40. In the lean enterprise model, what is the first step toward improving quality?

a. Establishing performance metrics.
b. Reviewing product design.
c. Understanding the expectations of the customer.
d. Identifying potential defects.

41. Time available divided by time available and time required is the Six Sigma ratio for:

a. productivity.
b. dependability.
c. customer satisfaction.
d. selectivity.

42. When prescriptions are being prepared, the labeling process begins at the same time as the medication is being packaged. However, the labeling does not take as long as the packaging. This difference in time does not add to the overall duration of the prescription-filling process. This is an example of:

a. just-in-time manufacturing.
b. slack time.
c. mistake proofing.
d. inherent process variation.

43. A hospital manager operates on the assumption that his employees will thrive when they are given responsibility and the opportunity to perform well. The manager's beliefs are aligned with:

    a. the theory of constraints.
    b. theory X.
    c. theory Y.
    d. theory Z.

44. Which of the following steps should be taken before QA activities begin?

    a. Responsibility should be shared.
    b. The principals should be informed.
    c. Resources should be pooled.
    d. The scope of involvement should be identified.

45. The protocol for ordering a medication should be:

    a. the same every time.
    b. customizable.
    c. adaptable to verbal or written situations.
    d. dependent on inventory.

46. Because the hospital is busy, an anesthesiologist is given less time than usual to examine the infusion device that will be delivering medication to a patient during surgery. The machine malfunctions and the doctors on hand must work feverishly to save the patient's life. This is an example of:

    a. active error.
    b. equipment error.
    c. system error.
    d. latent error.

47. In a typical hospital, approximately what percentage of errors is reported?

    a. Less than 5.
    b. Between 25 and 50.
    c. 75.
    d. Between 80 and 90.

48. A behavioral health specialist notices a particularly high number of restraint deaths at a facility. An analysis of the root causes of these events is most likely to indicate problems with:

    a. equipment.
    b. staff orientation and training.
    c. staffing levels.
    d. alarm systems.

49. A good meeting facilitator will:

    a. not need to ask very many questions.
    b. focus on process rather than content.
    c. refrain from offering suggestions.
    d. focus on content rather than process.

50. During the periods with the highest incoming workload, a laboratory that has not implemented lean practices is likely to have:

    a. substandard lead time performance.
    b. diminished productivity.
    c. false positives.
    d. selective engagement errors.

51. As much as possible, medications should be standardized. However, when this is impossible, it is important to:

    a. assume that side-effects will occur.
    b. warn clinicians about the potential for overdose.
    c. only use them as a last resort.
    d. differentiate them clearly.

52. Individual instruction on clinical governance is most effective when:

    a. it is delivered to a group.
    b. it is delivered before a performance review.
    c. it is combined with targeted training.
    d. it is targeted at new employees.

53. When establishing an incentive program for employees, the critical-to-quality parameters should be:

    a. agreed upon by all participants.
    b. attainable and significant.
    c. determined while the program is underway.
    d. established by the senior administrator.

54. A hospital uses the same labels for all of its prescriptions, but these labels do not fit on the smallest container, so employees must cut and paste the labels in a special way in order to fill the prescription. This is an example of:

    a. overproduction.
    b. queuing.
    c. work-in-progress.
    d. extra processing.

55. The discharge department of a hospital is at optimal efficiency when it completes the discharge process:

    a. more often than customer requests occur.
    b. at about the same rate as customer requests occur.
    c. less often than customer requests occur.
    d. twice as fast as customer requests occur.

56. When a hospital official notes that most errors are occurring at the "sharp end," he means that:

    a. they involve surgical tools or knives.
    b. they occur in clusters.
    c. they occur during the interactions between caregivers and patients.
    d. they are more likely to occur during busy periods.

57. During a meeting, the facilitator must intervene several times to stop disputes between participants. Is this appropriate?

a. Yes, but the facilitator should stay in the background unless the progress of the meeting is threatened.
b. Yes, the facilitator should rule in favor of one participant.
c. No, the facilitator should never intrude upon a meeting.
d. No, the facilitator should leave this duty to the chairperson.

58. Which of the following procedures is NOT a good way to mitigate injury?

a. Maintaining a ready supply of antidotes to high-risk medications.
b. Simulation training.
c. Programming equipment to shut off in the event of a crisis.
d. Requiring employees to practice crisis response.

59. The first and most important step in a disclosure conversation is:

a. assessing the patient's mood.
b. admitting error and apologizing.
c. discussing the root cause analysis.
d. compensating the patient.

60. Which of the following factors is NOT included in a calculation of risk priority number?

a. Severity of possible adverse effects.
b. Effectiveness of controls.
c. Likelihood of an adverse effect.
d. Cost of controls.

61. One consequence of the implementation of Lean Six Sigma practices in a hospital will be:

a. reduction in inventory.
b. the creation of systems for verifying orders.
c. reduction in staff.
d. reduction in manufacturing costs.

62. A program for assessing the validity of rolled throughput yield calculation is called:

a. composite clinical indication.
b. performance measure selection.
c. continuous quality management.
d. measurement systems analysis.

63. The general intent of the PDSA cycle is to:

a. optimize a process.
b. reduce bottlenecks.
c. incorporate new technology.
d. automate processes.

64. What are the three dimensions of quality in the most common framework for quality assessment?

a. Service, process, and mortality.
b. Structure, process, and outcomes.
c. Population, structure, and satisfaction.
d. Function, outcomes, and clinical status.

65. One common model for administrative meetings is for small groups to discuss specific problems and then join together in a:

a. process intervention.
b. confab.
c. colloquium.
d. plenary.

66. One characteristic of the SOAP model for medical records is:

a. the inclusion of both subjective and objective data.
b. the lack of a prognosis.
c. the focus on therapeutic intervention.
d. the absence of a differential diagnosis.

67. A top-level administrator is asked by a lower-level manager to lead a meeting of new employees. What should the administrator do first?

a. Review the notes from previous meetings.
b. Discuss the meeting participants with the manager.
c. Organize preliminary notes.
d. Compose an introductory statement.

68. A root cause analysis of inpatient suicides would be most likely to discover problems with:

a. staffing levels.
b. staff orientation.
c. the physical environment.
d. the availability of information.

69. A hospital's medication system is vast, and various elements of it fall within the purview of several different departments. One important step towards reducing errors in this system is to:

a. make each department responsible for the system as a whole.
b. have each department use the same self-assessment tools.
c. give a single person responsibility for overseeing the entire system.
d. simplify it.

70. After numerous staff meetings, a hospital administrator notices that one of his subordinates is an excellent content leader. Which of the following would the subordinate be most likely to do?

a. Suggest amendments to the meeting agenda.
b. Establish a tone of collegiality.
c. Enforce rules of conduct during the meeting.
d. Introduce new tools for examining data.

71. Why would a hospital include an APACHE III score on an analysis of the infection rate?

   a. To indicate trends related to age.
   b. To link infection with socioeconomic status.
   c. To find areas of resource waste.
   d. To establish the general likelihood of infection for patients with various conditions.

72. As part of the implementation of lean practices, a laboratory categorizes activities as either "value-add" or "non-value-add." What should be done with "non-value-add" activities?

   a. They should be minimized or, if possible, eliminated.
   b. They should be eliminated.
   c. They should be combined.
   d. They should be synchronized.

73. According to the Joint Commission, the primary cause of wrong-site surgery errors is:

   a. unusual patient characteristics.
   b. the necessity of multiple surgeries.
   c. communication failure.
   d. the presence of multiple surgeons.

74. A hospital uses infusion pumps to deliver intravenous medications. However, these pumps occasionally malfunction, so a nurse is assigned to periodically monitor their operation. Is this a good strategy?

   a. No, because it depends on the vigilance of one employee.
   b. No, because it will distract the nurse from her other duties.
   c. Yes, because it makes one person directly responsible.
   d. Yes, because it gives the nurse a clear directive.

75. One way to create useful alignment in an organization is to:

   a. base the assessment of each department on the same set of performance dimensions.
   b. have each employee report to a single manager.
   c. eliminate adverse drug events.
   d. organize interdepartmental meetings.

76. Which of the following is NOT mandatory in a generic dispensing program?

   a. Active ingredient must be the same.
   b. Chemical composition must be the same.
   c. Salt form must be the same.
   d. Dosage form must be the same.

77. If administrators are given a list of the variables that predict mortality for patients with a given condition, they should be able to:

   a. reduce the number of deaths.
   b. eliminate wasteful therapies.
   c. create a formula for the risk of death for each patient.
   d. reduce bottlenecks in the emergency room.

78. If an at-risk patient is left unattended and has an adverse response to medication, this is known as a(n):

    a. sentinel event.
    b. initiator.
    c. latent outcome.
    d. slip.

79. One important driver of customer dissatisfaction in health care over the past decade has been:

    a. the introduction of online services.
    b. the lack of communication between physicians and patients.
    c. the rise in income inequality.
    d. the improvement of customer care in other service industries.

80. Which of the following is most important?

    a. Patient satisfaction.
    b. Clinical satisfaction.
    c. Employee satisfaction.
    d. Patient, clinical, and employee satisfaction are equally important.

81. The minimum practical lead time for an analytical laboratory is:

    a. the release constraint test time for the microbiology lab.
    b. greater than the release constraint test time for the microbiology lab.
    c. less than the release constraint test time for the microbiology lab.
    d. unrelated to the release constraint test time for the microbiology lab

82. Which of the following contracts would be most appropriate when remodeling an old wing of a hospital?

    a. Formal contract.
    b. Time and materials contract.
    c. Cost reimbursement contract.
    d. Fixed price contract.

83. In the optimal decision-making process, the most time will be devoted to:

    a. framing the question.
    b. learning from feedback.
    c. drawing conclusions.
    d. gathering information.

84. In lean enterprise, which is the worst type of waste?

    a. Extra processing.
    b. Queuing.
    c. Transport.
    d. Overproduction.

85. Team paralysis is NOT a common result of:

a. rigid adherence to meeting protocol.
b. lack of familiarity with subject matter.
c. the failure to build consensus.
d. an overabundance of options.

86. A set of key measures that is used to judge progress is known as a(n):

a. performance factor.
b. dashboard.
c. independent variable.
d. benchmark.

87. Volatility in nursing workload is less likely to be reported than other sources of waste because:

a. nurses are unlikely to complain.
b. it can only be perceived through the use of advanced metrics.
c. it is less observable.
d. it takes place infrequently.

88. A hospital's automated pharmacy program will not fill a prescription unless the patient's allergy information has been entered. This is an example of:

a. constraint.
b. natural mapping.
c. affordance.
d. standardization.

89. The frequency of errors in a particular process would best be displayed in a(n):

a. matrix diagram.
b. pareto chart.
c. affinity diagram.
d. histogram.

90. One disadvantage of using separate scorecards for financial and customer satisfaction data is that:

a. administrators are likely to overvalue the financial information.
b. employees will become confused.
c. there is likely to be more resource waste.
d. it requires special training.

91. The most common source of the goal statement for a tree diagram is:

a. an affinity diagram.
b. the root cause identified by an interrelationship digraph.
c. an assignment.
d. a histogram.

92. One of the consequences of successful application of the theory of constraints is:

  a. major system changes.
  b. fewer employees.
  c. the creation of new constraints.
  d. capital improvements.

93. Most quality problems in healthcare are the result of:

  a. lack of compassion.
  b. lack of resources.
  c. disorganization.
  d. ignorance.

94. The system limits of a process typically are based on the average and standard deviation of the:

  a. yield and error rate.
  b. duration and validity.
  c. yield and duration.
  d. validity and yield.

95. A hospital administrator wants to determine how changes in resource allocation would affect total profit. By manipulating a variable, for instance the number of nurses assigned to a floor of the hospital, the administrator can calculate the difference in profit. The administrator is performing a:

  a. sensitivity analysis.
  b. risk analysis.
  c. force field analysis.
  d. decision analysis.

96. Over the past three decades, medical knowledge and technology have:

  a. expanded at a slow rate.
  b. expanded at an exponential rate.
  c. both expanded and declined at different times.
  d. declined at a slow rate.

97. It has been determined that a hospital's blood transfusions are 99.7 percent error-free. Which function can be used to determine the number of blood transfusions that are likely to be performed before an error is made?

  a. Binomial distribution.
  b. Poisson distribution.
  c. Negative binomial distribution.
  d. Multinomial distribution.

98. An increase in chronic conditions is one consequence of:

  a. more complicated intervention strategies.
  b. advances in medical technology.
  c. greater population density.
  d. longer life expectancy.

99. In healthcare, the most common adjustment to the traditional balanced scorecard is the:

a. focus on financial performance.
b. extra emphasis on patient results and customer satisfaction.
c. elimination of business operations.
d. use of advanced metrics.

100. Which of the following is a reactive system?

a. Questionnaires.
b. Market research.
c. Information obtained from customer complaints.
d. Interviews with customers.

101. The "four bads" associated with drug-related morbidity are:

a. bad drugs, bad doctors, bad pharmacists, and bad patients.
b. bad drugs, bad patients, bad luck, and bad doctors.
c. bad drugs, bad pharmacists, bad nurses, and bad luck.
d. bad drugs, bad patients, bad prescribing, and bad luck.

102. A quality improvement team wants to construct a simple chart that will depict how institutional spending and time are applied to a set of basic tasks. This chart will take the form of a:

a. T-shaped matrix.
b. L-shaped matrix.
c. X-shaped matrix.
d. Y-shaped matrix.

103. If the load and the mix of a testing laboratory are leveled, the result will be:

a. an increase in capacity.
b. a reduction in cost.
c. an increase in capacity and/or a reduction in cost.
d. an increase in capacity or a reduction in cost.

104. One difference between evidence-based practice and research utilization is that:

a. research utilization takes into account the preferences of the patient.
b. research utilization relies on only one study.
c. evidence-based practice is based on tradition.
d. evidence-based practice incorporates the ideas of opinion leaders.

105. Which of the following is NOT one of the basic components of an optimization model?

a. Constraints.
b. Objective function.
c. Variable inputs.
d. Price information.

106. At present, the best way to improve the delivery of accurate and useful information about medication would be to:

   a. create a universal database of patient records.
   b. improve the time it takes pharmacies to deliver medicine.
   c. give patients access to their lab reports.
   d. encourage pharmacists to visit nursing stations regularly.

107. In general, how many steps should a failure modes and effects analysis take in each direction?

   a. 1.
   b. 2.
   c. 5.
   d. 10.

108. Team members begin to reach consensus on the rules for operation during the stage known as:

   a. storming.
   b. forming.
   c. norming.
   d. recognition.

109. Which of the following is a characteristic of a high-performing group?

   a. More advocacy than inquiry.
   b. More internal than external focus.
   c. More skepticism than optimism.
   d. A blend of internal focus and external review.

110. Which component of decision-making typically receives much less time than it deserves?

   a. Framing.
   b. Gathering information.
   c. Drawing conclusions.
   d. Voting.

111. Which of the following is NOT a goal of quality circles?

   a. To improve customer relations.
   b. To develop new services.
   c. To improve job satisfaction.
   d. To maximize employee potential.

112. In the most efficient labs, each technician:

   a. can only complete a single task.
   b. performs every task.
   c. can perform every task, but usually performs only one.
   d. rotates between tasks on a daily basis.

113. A health care facility has eleven wheelchairs. The likelihood that a wheelchair will be available when needed can be calculated with a(n):

a. binomial distribution.
b. multinomial distribution.
c. factorial.
d. effects analysis.

114. When developing quality standards, the best source of information is:

a. trade publications.
b. the facility scorecard.
c. prior performance measures.
d. external benchmarking data.

115. Which of the following is NOT a primary goal of lean enterprise?

a. Improve quality.
b. Stabilize total costs.
c. Eliminate waste.
d. Reduce lead time.

116. Why is it important to use customized benchmarks?

a. Administrators may not release comprehensive data.
b. Customer satisfaction is the most important measure of success.
c. External factors may differentiate otherwise similar organizations.
d. Customization eliminates resource waste.

117. At the beginning of a planning meeting, the participants are asked to make a list of their priorities. These lists are then compiled, and an overall list of priorities is created. This process is known as:

a. nominal group technique.
b. diversion and conversion.
c. force field analysis.
d. multi-voting.

118. Which of the following is NOT one of the operational measurements emphasized by the theory of constraints?

a. Throughput.
b. Operating expense.
c. Inventory.
d. Net profit.

119. A hospital experiences very infrequent problems with infusion equipment. The best statistical distribution model for examining these errors would be the:

a. binomial distribution.
b. Poisson distribution.
c. normal distribution.
d. multinomial distribution.

120. The most common and effective style of checklist for hospital employees is:

a. standardized and rarely updated.
b. requires detailed responses.
c. only required for new employees.
d. designed to prompt a response of "yes" to almost every question.

121. A meeting facilitator notices that the team has a tendency towards groupthink. What is one structural way to correct this problem?

a. Meet late in the day.
b. Meet more often.
c. Break the group down into smaller subgroups.
d. Have comments submitted in writing.

122. Employee incentive programs should emphasize:

a. adherence to established protocols.
b. excellent results.
c. improved cost savings.
d. reduction in adverse events.

123. When assessing an emergency room, the best strategy for data collection is:

a. cluster sampling.
b. continuous sampling.
c. matched random sampling.
d. accidental sampling.

124. Which of the following is NOT one of the four elements of a health service microsystem?

a. A clear and identifiable population of patients.
b. An environment in which self-assessment information can be obtained.
c. A broad collection of health-care providers, support personnel, and private contractors.
d. Well though-out work processes.

125. What is one advantage of a voluntary error reporting system over a mandatory error reporting system?

a. Mandatory systems are only targeted at very narrow areas of practice.
b. Voluntary systems eliminate the need for communication between healthcare organizations.
c. Voluntary systems elicit more reports from front-line practitioners.
d. Mandatory systems discourage the reporting of non-fatal errors.

126. The main difference between the Taguchi model of service provision and the traditional model is that:

a. the Taguchi model identifies waste any time a process varies from its target.
b. the traditional model is less forgiving of error.
c. the Taguchi model is only applicable to manufacturing processes.
d. the traditional model requires an organization with at least fifty employees.

127. An administrative team is using an interrelationship digraph to examine the problem of nursing workload volatility. What will the team do after making a list of the factors that influence this issue?

a. Confer with an expert.
b. Tabulate the data.
c. Identify root causes.
d. Draw relationship arrows between the factors.

128. To deal with volatile workloads, a laboratory creates a fast track for samples that need to be processed immediately. One common result of this strategy is that:

a. average lead times will be reduced.
b. the laboratory will stop having bottlenecks.
c. technicians will become confused.
d. the portion of samples placed in the fast track will steadily increase.

129. Which of the following diagrams is appropriate for categorizing the needs of customers?

a. Kano model.
b. Histogram.
c. Flow chart.
d. Matrix diagram.

130. The most important characteristic of the controls in a case-control study is that they are:

a. drawn from a random pool of patients.
b. identical to the cases in every respect except for the presence of the targeted condition.
c. available for frequent observation.
d. literate.

131. When a hospital administration decides on strategy, this information should be shared with:

a. employees, patients, and the community.
b. employees only.
c. employees and patients only.
d. no one.

132. When conducting an audit of a large department, an administrator will likely apply the central limit theorem. What does this mean?

a. He will average all of the data from the department.
b. He will focus his efforts on the departmental leadership.
c. He will assume that a sample is representative of the department as a whole.
d. He will compare the department's performance to ISO 9001 standards.

133. One common problem in labs with low turnover is:

a. excessive slack time.
b. narrow specialization by technicians.
c. failure to adapt.
d. confrontations between management and technicians.

134. Frequent benchmarking is important in lean service because:

a. it boosts employee morale.
b. it prevents an organization from failing to react to external changes.
c. it eliminates employee waste.
d. it reduces adverse drug events.

135. Root cause analyses most often reveal that mistakes are the result of:

a. a series of small errors.
b. a single miscalculation.
c. a culture of incompetence.
d. bad actors.

136. Which of the following is the strongest basis for practice?

a. Systematic reviews of randomized clinical trials.
b. Descriptive studies.
c. Qualitative studies.
d. Opinion leaders.

137. Research suggests that people make fewer errors when they:

a. perform several tasks at once.
b. work creatively.
c. work individually.
d. work in a team.

138. A brief analysis of interventions for stroke is likely to be relatively unhelpful because:

a. most stroke victims die.
b. stroke victims tend to be very old.
c. research has yet to discover an effective standard treatment.
d. strokes are likely to be accompanied by other conditions.

139. Hospitals pay special attention to blood transfusions because:

a. they are easy to monitor and verify.
b. they are rare.
c. they are responsible for the largest percentage of malpractice suits.
d. they are complicated and dangerous.

140. The main difference between a dashboard and a scorecard is that:

a. a dashboard is only to be viewed by senior administrators.
b. a scorecard includes performance measures from multiple departments.
c. a dashboard only includes one measure of performance.
d. a scorecard describes past performance, while a dashboard depicts performance in real time.

Answer Key and Explanations for Test #1

1. A: According to the Institute of Medicine, the three domains of quality care are customization, safety, and interventions consistent with the latest medical findings. These domains provide the basic structure for the IOM's recommendations about quality care originally presented in the groundbreaking book *To Err Is Human*. Government regulation is an essential part of quality care, but it is not a domain in itself. Instead, the IOM recommends that healthcare facilities work with government agencies to develop fair but efficient regulatory policies that protect practitioners and patients alike.

2. C: Independent contractors are the group least likely to report errors. In part, this is because they have the least personal interest in the success of the health care facility. Also, an independent contractor is more likely to view his employment as tenuous, and is therefore more nervous about admitting mistakes. A system that explicitly avoids punishing those who report will improve the incidence of error reporting among independent contractors.

3. B: Abuse is not one of the types of quality problems identified by the Institute of Medicine's National Roundtable on Health Care Quality. Misuse, overuse, and underuse are the three most common problems; they also represent three sources of waste in health care. The National Roundtable on Health Care Quality was significant because it asserted that the provision of health care services can be assessed with scientific precision. This was a major step towards incorporating business and manufacturing productivity systems in health care.

4. B: In behavioral health, the most important sentinel event for root cause analysis is death. A sentinel event is any adverse occurrence that is outside the range of the normal progression of the diagnosed illness. In other words, death can only be a sentinel event when it occurs in patients who are not expected to die. In cases where death is not considered likely, it is usually the most important sentinel event, because it is the one that most urgently requires investigation and prevention. The term *sentinel event* was popularized by the Joint Commission.

5. D: It is easy to conduct a survey of medication-related errors because prescription drug use is common and well documented. For this reason, there is a vast literature on the subject. However, many other types of error remain relatively unexplored. For instance, latent errors, like those related to poor training or improper calibration of equipment, are much less likely to be analyzed. Nevertheless, it is important to continue analyzing medication-related errors, both because they are quite common and because they are dangerous and costly. There is currently a movement to establish a standardized medication-error reporting system that will enable the compilation of statistics on a larger scale.

6. A: In a successful lean healthcare facility, the largest costs related to quality will be incurred by preventive efforts. Indeed, a lean facility is likely to spend much more than another facility on prevention. A lean facility saves money by reducing errors and eliminating waste. Moreover, prevention programs in a lean facility tend to be more efficient and targeted. Over time, a lean healthcare facility may be able to phase out certain elements of prevention.

7. B: The best time to discuss the results of a meeting exit survey is at the beginning of the next meeting. This gives the team members the best opportunity to apply the results of the survey immediately. A facilitator should use an exit survey to improve the protocol of meetings. It is best for these surveys to remain anonymous so that respondents will feel comfortable being honest. Email is not a good medium for exit surveys because it creates a permanent and traceable record and therefore discourages honesty.

8. C: Whenever possible, medication orders should be by dose. This is the most important variable related to medication, and the one which has the most relevance to the products actually used by the patient. Medication orders that are classified by weight, volume, or strength are often confusing to pharmacists. Moreover, several different unit systems (e.g., metric or SI) may be used, so there is a greater risk of error. To reduce the possibility of mistakes, healthcare facilities should standardize the protocol for medication orders.

9. A: The best explanation for the relatively slow introduction of lean practices into medical laboratories is that the variability and complexity of the samples in the laboratory is much higher than in a manufacturing environment. In laboratories, it is common for a huge number of slightly different samples to be processed. A simple assembly line approach to laboratory processes is rarely successful. However, there are striking analogies between manufacturing and laboratory work, and laboratories can drastically improve efficiency by adopting lean practices. Contrary to the beliefs of some, lean practices do not discourage innovation. Instead, they enable laboratories to handle greater volume and diversity without sacrificing quality.

10. B: A simple but effective way for managers to obtain the support of team members is to ask for it. Unfortunately, many assertive managers feel that openly requesting buy-in from team members is a sign of weakness. What they do not realize is that the members of a team are more likely to respond positively to a leader who they believe is humble and capable of admitting that he needs help. Threats and coercion only antagonize subordinates. In a healthcare facility, team leaders are likely to be dealing with healthy egos. The best way to elicit the support of confident and independent doctors and nurses is to request it directly.

11. D: A delay in discharging patients is likely to cause recurrent bottlenecks in admissions from the emergency room and surgical wards and in the filling of prescriptions. Indeed, the negative consequences of discharge delays may include the creation of other bottlenecks. It is important to recognize that inefficiencies in one area of service provision can cause inefficiencies in many other areas. A bottleneck occurs when there are not enough resources available to perform all of the functions necessary at a given time. Discharge delays waste time, money, and resources.

12. D: A quality assessment program should not include rare conditions that have a small effect on mortality or morbidity. Such conditions have a limited bearing on the overall success of care. There is a general agreement as to which conditions are appropriate for inclusion in a quality assessment program. A condition should meet five criteria. First, it should either be common or have a significant effect on morbidity or mortality. Second, there should be scientific evidence that there are treatments effective at preventing or mitigating the effects of the condition. Third, it should be established that improvement in the quality of treatment for the condition will improve overall health. Fourth, the condition should have cost-effective interventions. Finally, the interventions for the condition should be susceptible to significant influence by health care providers.

13. C: When a doctor fails to administer an indicated test and the patient has an adverse result, the doctor has committed a diagnostic error. A diagnostic error is committed whenever a condition is misidentified or an indicated test is not performed. A diagnostic error can result in even more errors in the future. A preventive error is a mistaken approach to avoiding a condition, while a treatment error is a mistake related to the resolution of a condition. A communication error may occur between two service providers or between a service provider and a patient.

14. B: The best time for chairing is at the beginning of a meeting. In most cases, the facilitator and the chairperson of the meeting are two different people. The chairperson is responsible for reviewing the minutes from the previous meeting and eliciting feedback from team members. A facilitator may be charged with organizing and moderating discussion, but the introduction to the meeting is typically conducted by the chairperson. In many situations, it is appropriate to rotate the chairing duties.

15. C: Tradition does not contribute to evidence-based practice in healthcare. The evidence-based practice movement consists of a renewed emphasis on scientific rigor and empirical data. The preferences of patients are considered, but the primary determinant of intervention and therapy is the evidence from research studies and the experience of practitioners. Traditional methods of therapy may be investigated to determine their efficacy, but they are not used for sentimental or cultural reasons. In addition to clinical expertise, evidence, and patient preferences, evidence-based practice devises therapies based on patient history and the availability of resources.

16. A: SIPOC (suppliers, inputs, process, outputs, customers) is different from the other three acronyms, which are sequential programs for quality improvement. SIPOC, on the other hand, is a form of diagram that enables Six Sigma practitioners to identify the important components of process improvement. DMAIC (define, measure, analyze, improve, control) is a general structure for eliminating defects. Similarly, PDCA (plan, do, check, act) and PDSA (plan, do, study, act) are structures for the improvement of processes.

17. A: In the perfect lean enterprise, delivery to the customer is instantaneous. Of course, instantaneous delivery is rarely possible. Nevertheless, the strategy of lean enterprise is to examine all of the ways in which service provision deviates from the ideal, and then to minimize these ways as much as possible. A lean healthcare facility will never attain instantaneous delivery, but it can continually improve by aiming for this standard. Of the other answer choices, it is true that lean enterprises often offer customizable delivery, but this is not a necessary condition of lean enterprise.

18. B: A presentation on the basic structures and processes of clinical governance would be most useful for the organization as a whole. Such a general presentation would really only be effective as an introduction for the entire organization. Other presentations, such as those delivered to small teams, the directorate, or individual employees, will need to be more targeted and specific. It is a good idea to introduce the basic concepts of clinical governance to the entire organization because the transition to this method of management often entails drastic change.

19. A: A hospital-wide set of professional standards is important because it reduces the waste of time and resources. As much as possible, healthcare facilities should standardize professional behavior in every department in order to eliminate confusion and reduce inefficient behavior. In some cases, the adoption of universal professional standards will reduce the need for communication, but this is not a necessary consequence. Similarly, it may be that standardization will decrease the number of bottlenecks, though again, this is not inevitable.

20. C: One disadvantage of the visioning strategy for setting goals is that the group must have at least six members for it to be feasible. In visioning, team members gather in groups of two and create lists of possible solutions to a problem. Each person then switches partners and shares his list. This process is repeated at least one more time, though in some visioning exercises team members partner up with seven or eight different people. Visioning is effective because it allows individual team members to interact with a large number of peers within a one-on-one setting that encourages effective communication.

21. C: Before conducting a safety audit in an emergency department, an administrator must first obtain a written set of safety standards. This is necessary so that the administrator can compare his observations to the established protocol. The general purpose of a safety audit is to identify areas in which the department deviates from standard procedure. In order to perform an effective audit, the administrator needs to have a general familiarity with the rules that his employees follow.

22. C: In the given situation, the best question for the facilitator to ask would be, "Were you feeling irritated during the meeting?" This phrasing is appropriate because it does not make assumptions about the participant's feelings. It may be that the participant was not irritated, or was irritated by something unrelated to the meeting. In any case, the facilitator should not make any suppositions without first talking to the participant.

23. A: The process chain in a laboratory is particularly subject to variability. In most medical laboratories, there is a great degree of volatility in the number of samples. This can be devastating to efficiency, particularly as it can create delays or necessitate the hiring of extra employees. Many laboratories are adopting lean manufacturing strategies to reduce delays and smooth out the variability of operations.

24. D: Research suggests that the largest proportion of adverse effects attributable to negligence occur in the emergency room, where the volatile workload and elevated stress level is most conducive to negligent acts. However, there are steps that can be taken to reduce these adverse events. Standardization and comprehensive training can diminish, though not eliminate, the incidence of adverse events related to negligence.

25. D: Verbal orders are the source of the most medication errors. Automatic orders, on the other hand, are responsible for the least medication errors. Verbal orders are more likely to be misunderstood or forgotten. Even though many doctors have notoriously bad handwriting, written prescriptions are still likely to be filled correctly. It is best to automate prescriptions as much as possible, and then to standardize the process for verbal orders. For instance, many facilities reduce errors by mandating that verbal prescriptions always be measured in metric units.

26. A: "What do you hope to accomplish in the meeting?" is not one of the typical questions in a force-field analysis. A force-field analysis is a retrospective rather than a prospective look at meeting structure and organization. In other words, it is a tool used to review what has happened in the past rather than to plan for the future. Force field analysis is based on the idea that progress can be made by enumerating the forces that contribute to or hinder the achievement of goals. Facilitators often use this technique to streamline meetings.

27. B: The definitive proof of the success of a regulation program is a decreased need for inspections. Ultimately, the presence of a comprehensive and effective regulatory system means that rules are followed without enforcement being required as often. The other answer choices represent frequent positive consequences of effective regulation, but are not necessarily indicative of regulatory success. The initial costs of implementing a regulatory program can be high, but become cost effective over time.

28. C: In the scenario described here, the most likely cause is that the drugs come in similar packaging. Errors resulting from similar packaging are surprisingly common in healthcare facilities. As a result, many facilities take specific steps to label or otherwise differentiate such medications. Although it can be valuable to have standardized packaging for drugs, there must also be a clear and universal system for differentiation.

29. D: One advantage of the kaizen approach to DMAIC implementation is that it is accomplished in about a week. During this period, almost all other operations must be suspended as employees devote themselves entirely to learning the new system. There are a few different systems for implementing a DMAIC (define, measure, analyze, improve, control) program for process improvement. The appropriate implementation system depends on the situation. However, the success of the kaizen approach helps refute the argument that Six Sigma is costly and time-consuming to implement.

30. D: The practice of waiting for a certain number of samples before commencing a test run results in longer lead times. In any process, lead time is the interval between the first step and the delivery of results. It stands to reason, then, that intentional delays in sample processing will create longer lead times. Many laboratories feel that it is more efficient to wait for a larger batch of samples before conducting a run. Lean practitioners, however, recommend that samples be processed as soon as they are ready. Reduction in lead time contributes to greater efficiency and the ability to handle larger volume.

31. C: A whole systems approach to clinical governance is important because changes must be applied at all levels of the organization. Men and women involved in clinical governance have to look at the big picture, which means that they must consider all of the elements and interrelationships of the healthcare facility. It may be that consideration of the healthcare facility as a whole will lead to the isolation of particular areas of concern, but this is not a necessary consequence. Taking the whole systems approach to clinical governance requires more than one week; indeed, it is an orientation that lasts for the entire life of the healthcare facility.

32. C: In this scenario, the prescription should not count towards the pharmacy's yield. In lean service provision, only those processes that are completed without the necessity of reworking or repair are considered as a part of yield. The goal of lean service implementation is to improve yields by reducing errors and defects. Mistakes due to bad handwriting are common in healthcare, which has led many facilities to standardize notation and introduce labeling or bar-coding systems. Such errors do not need to be reported to the FDA.

33. C: In this scenario, a reorganization of the hospital hierarchy should minimize the manager's span of control. The span of control is the number of subordinates who report directly to a single supervisor. Over the past few decades, a general trend towards flattening organizational structures has increased the average span of control. Whereas, in the past, 10 was considered the largest number of employees that could be effectively supervised by a single manager, now it is common for a single manager to be responsible for the work of dozens of employees. As a result, ineffective leadership has increased.

34. A: Hospitals that implement computerized provider order entry (CPOE) almost always see a decline in medication errors. CPOE is a standard program for automating medical instructions. Implementation of a CPOE program diminishes errors related to faulty transcription or unclear handwriting. These programs also simplify inventory and decrease delays in order completion. Perhaps more importantly, the implementation of a CPOE program in large facilities enables employees to give and receive orders without being in physical proximity to one another.

35. A: In a traditional meeting, the timekeeper and the minute taker roles are filled by different people every time. Rotating these positions enables every member of the group to participate. It is a good idea to have these functions performed by two different people because they can be somewhat distracting and time-consuming. Establishing a regular rotation for timekeeping and minute taking is one way to improve teamwork and cooperation in a group.

36. D: An adverse drug reaction is defined as harm caused to a patient as a result of the administration of a drug. It may manifest as a presentation of a negative symptom or simply a reduced effectiveness of other therapies. An unforeseen side effect or a drug interaction may or may not be harmful to the patient. Harm that occurs during or after a drug administration would be better identified as an adverse drug event, unless it can be shown that the medication was the cause.

37. B: This sort of decision should be made by voting. Relatively insignificant decisions should not be allowed to take up a large amount of time. The process of building a consensus or brainstorming on a trivial subject, such as the one described here, would be a waste of resources. At the same time, it is always productive to give managers a voice rather than to make decisions by decree. A simple vote will quickly dispatch this unimportant issue so that the group can move on to more important subjects.

38. D: Confronted by excessive WIP levels, many laboratories take the unhelpful step of installing new technology. Too often, laboratory managers assume that new technology will solve their problems without considering just how this will occur. Before installing new technology, a laboratory manager would be wise to run a DMAIC program to identify areas for improvement.

39. A: When establishing a clinical governance training program for the directorate, it is useful to align the subject matter with the specific tasks of the audience. Because it can be assumed that members of the directorate will already be familiar with the general concepts of clinical governance, it is much more effective to choose training programs for narrow and specific tasks. However, it is not efficient to customize instruction for each member of the directorate. Case studies are an essential part of clinical governance training.

40. A: In the lean enterprise model, the first step toward improving quality is establishing performance metrics. These metrics are the scale on which progress will be measured. They should be appropriate and general so that performance can be compared between departments and with other successful organizations. The other answer choices represent essential steps in lean enterprise, but they are based on solid performance metrics.

41. B: Time available divided by time available and time required is the Six Sigma ratio for dependability. In Six Sigma, dependability is the degree to which a process or product is available when it is needed. The implementation of Six Sigma practices requires products with a high degree of dependability because processes need to be completed as quickly as possible. One of the major contributions of Six Sigma and other productivity philosophies has been the application of scientific principles and formulas to manufacturing and the provision of services.

42. B: This scenario is an example of slack time. Slack time is the interval between the first and last times at which a process can be completed without delaying the overall project. In this case, some slack time is inevitable. The packaging process will always take a little longer than the labeling process. As a result, the duration of this step of the process has a minimum duration equal to the time required for packaging. Almost every system has some slack time, but it should be diminished as much as possible.

43. C: The hospital manager's beliefs are aligned with theory Y. Theory Y is the management philosophy that believes employees will thrive when they are given responsibility and the chance to innovate. Theory Y amounts to an optimistic view of human nature. Theory X, on the other hand, is a more skeptical management orientation. Adherents of theory X believe that people are lazy by nature, and will only perform their duties competently if they are monitored closely. Most managers blend these two theories in their professional practice.

44. D: Before QA activities begin, the scope of involvement should be identified. The scope of involvement is the entire set of materials, processes, and people that are required for a project. It is impossible to understand fully the influences on a project's success without first identifying the scope of involvement. Quality assurance requires a systematic approach to identifying the scope of involvement. Responsibility and resources should not necessarily be shared before the initiation of quality assurance activities. On the contrary, one hallmark of successful QA is clear designation of responsibility, in particular for resources.

45. A: The protocol for ordering medication should be the same every time. Medication errors are among the most common and most preventable in a healthcare facility. One way to reduce these errors is to standardize the prescription process. Many healthcare facilities achieve a drastic reduction in medication errors by forbidding verbal orders. In any case, the protocol for ordering a medication should not be customizable, as this is likely to create confusion and lead to error.

46. D: This scenario is an example of latent error. A latent error is one made during setup or programming that creates negative consequences in the future. These sorts of errors are very difficult to identify, because they take place at a time far removed from the adverse events. In this instance, a latent error is present both in the malfunction of the machine and the short amount of time allotted to the anesthesiologist. Many times, it takes a combination of multiple latent errors to create an adverse event. Hospital managers are responsible for taking a detached and broad view of operations to identify and eliminate the sources of latent error.

47. A: In a typical hospital, less than five percent of errors are reported. Many hospital managers are surprised by this statistic, because the number of reported errors can seem large. However, healthcare facilities often have unclear or relaxed reporting policies. Part-time employees and independent contractors are much less likely to report errors. Unfortunately, the failure to report errors has negative consequences far beyond the point at which the specific error occurs. The best healthcare facilities establish mandatory error-reporting programs with an emphasis on being nonjudgmental and accepting of inevitable human error.

48. B: An analysis of the root causes of an abnormally high number of restraint deaths is most likely to indicate problems with staff orientation and training. Equipment, staffing levels, and alarm systems can also be culpable in restraint deaths, but problems with orientation and training are much more likely. Restraint equipment has been designed to be very safe when it is used correctly. When used improperly, restraint equipment can be deadly. It should be noted that most root cause analyses indicate problems in multiple areas.

49. B: A good meeting facilitator will focus on process rather than content. Indeed, a facilitator need not even be familiar with the subject of the meeting to do his job well. No matter the content, the structure and administration of the meeting will proceed along similar lines. The other answer choices represent poor choices for a meeting facilitator. The facilitator should always ask a great many questions before leaving a meeting. He should also offer suggestions whenever appropriate. With experience, a facilitator learns when to interject and when to stay on the periphery.

50. A: During the periods with the highest incoming workload, a laboratory that has not implemented lean practices is likely to have substandard lead time performance. Lead time is the full interval required to complete a process or fill an order. Longer lead times are considered substandard. Productivity, on the other hand, may be higher than normal during the periods with the highest incoming workload, as the laboratory is engaged in constant processing. A big spike in productivity is not necessarily a good thing, however, because it may indicate that the lab is not making the best use of its down time. In an ideal scenario, there is little difference in productivity or lead time regardless of incoming workload. This is known as smoothing out the workload.

51. D: When it is impossible for medications to be standardized, it is important to differentiate them clearly. Many medications have similar packaging and labeling, and so should be clearly distinguished in order to reduce medication errors. Hospitals and healthcare facilities often use color-coding or electronic tags to differentiate similar-looking medications.

52. C: Individual instruction on clinical governance is most effective when it is combined with targeted training. Clinical governance is a comprehensive approach to improving the quality of healthcare. It is a vast and complex subject that requires a great deal of employee education. Clinical governance training should not be tied to performance review, nor should it be delivered exclusively to new employees. It requires ongoing attention at all levels of the organization.

53. B: When establishing an incentive program for employees, the critical-to-quality parameters should be attainable and significant. The critical-to-quality parameters are targets that, when attained, will result in superior performance. Employee incentive programs should always focus on task performance rather than results. After all, employees can only be held responsible for doing their jobs according to prescribed protocol. If the results of their efforts are negative, then the protocols should be examined. Although the critical-to-quality parameters should not be determined by a democratic process, neither should they be established solely by a senior administrator. Instead, they should be the result of a clear-eyed determination of the most important and variable tasks in every process.

54. D: This scenario is an example of extra processing. Extra processing is anathema to the philosophy of lean. Whenever a lean manager spots a situation like the one in this example, he will immediately work to resolve it. In this case, the hospital would be wise to adopt a labeling system that is appropriate for all of its containers. In addition to the obvious creation of more work, the extra processing described here may encourage medication errors.

55. B: The discharge department of a hospital is at optimal efficiency when it completes the discharge progress at about the same rate as customer requests occur. Discharges cannot occur more often than customer requests. If discharges occur less frequently than customer requests, the discharge department is inefficient. It can be difficult to optimize a discharge department, as discharges tend to occur in clusters, which can be difficult to predict.

56. C: When a hospital official notes that most errors are occurring at the "sharp end," he means that they occur during the interactions between caregivers and patients. The phrases "sharp end" and "blunt end" are used by quality management professionals to describe areas of practice. The "sharp end" is all of the operations that involve direct contact with the patient, client, or customer. The "blunt end" is all of the behind-the-scenes actions that take place outside of the awareness of the patient, client, or customer. Although patients are more likely to notice errors at the sharp end, there are significantly more errors committed at the blunt end.

57. A: It is appropriate for a facilitator to intervene when the progress of the meeting is threatened. After all, it is the job of a facilitator to maintain forward momentum and adhere to the meeting protocol. In some cases, however, disputes between meeting participants can be fruitful and should be allowed to continue. But more often than not, confrontations only serve to alienate participants.

58. C: Programming equipment to shut off in the event of a crisis is not a good way to mitigate injury. Equipment should be programmed to default to the least-harmful setting, but in many cases shutting off is as harmful as operating incorrectly. For instance, a respirator should never default to an "off" position. All of the other answer choices represent excellent strategies for mitigating injury.

59. B: The first and most important step in a disclosure conversation is admitting an error and apologizing. The wisdom of apologizing has long been a source of contention in healthcare circles. For many years, it was widely thought that an apology would leave the practitioner vulnerable to malpractice suits. However, recent legislation has established that an apology does not mean an admission of negligence or malpractice. It is now considered prudent to mollify a potentially confrontational patient or client by issuing a sincere apology.

60. D: The cost of controls is not included in a calculation of risk priority number. A risk priority number, or RPN, is an objective picture of the importance of a particular danger to performance. It is calculated by rating on a scale from 1 to 10 the severity of each possible adverse effect (where 10 is the most severe), the likelihood of each of these effects (where 10 is the most certain to occur), and the effectiveness of possible controls (where 1 is the most effective), and then multiplying these three numbers.

61. A: One consequence of the implementation of Lean Six Sigma practices in a hospital will be a reduction in inventory. Indeed, reduced inventory is one of the fundamental goals of Lean Six Sigma. The developers of this organizational philosophy assert that there are numerous costs associated with maintaining a large inventory. Essentially, they believe that it is impossible to operate at peak efficiency while maintaining a large store of products and resources. Although many people believe that the implementation of Lean Six Sigma practices will lead to reductions in staff and manufacturing costs, this is not necessarily the case.

62. D: A program for assessing the validity of rolled throughput yield calculation is called measurement systems analysis (MSA). MSA is used to evaluate many of the metrics used in business. All sorts of factors can influence the equipment and methodology used to measure performance. Because advanced productivity systems like Six Sigma and lean depend on accurate and detailed statistics, effective measurement systems analysis is essential.

63. A: The general intent of the PDSA cycle is to optimize a new process. This cycle has four steps: plan, do, study, and act. It is sometimes referred to as PDCA (plan, do, check, act) or the Deming cycle. The first step of this cycle is to identify the targets that must be met in order to achieve output goals. The next step is to implement the new processes, often on a small scale. The third step is to measure the performance of the new processes and compare it with the expected results. Finally, the last step is to determine areas for improvement.

64. B: In the most common framework for quality assessment, the three dimensions of quality are structure, process, and outcomes. The structure of care is the basic elements of the population and the health care provider. Care can only succeed to the extent that the structure allows. Elements of structure include the characteristics of the community, healthcare organization, population, and healthcare provider. Process is the dynamic act of care provision. It includes both technical and interpersonal excellence, because quality care requires not only competence but also responsiveness to the emotional needs of patients. Finally, outcomes are the full range of results from care. Clinical status and mortality are outcomes, but so is patient satisfaction.

65. D: One common model for administrative meetings is for small groups to discuss specific problems and then gather in a plenary. This model is also popular for conferences. A plenary session usually includes a general summary of what has been discussed in the small-group meetings, with an opportunity for participants to ask questions and offer comments.

66. A: One characteristic of the SOAP model for medical records is the inclusion of both subjective and objective data. The SOAP model is a common method of organizing medical information. The subjective part of the record includes the patient's presenting complaint, symptoms, and any information obtained in the interview. The objective component consists of the results of the physical examination and any additional tests (e.g., blood test, MRI). The assessment is the clinician's diagnosis. Finally, the plan is the set of recommended treatments.

67. B: The administrator's first step should be to discuss the meeting participants with the manager. This discussion will inform and organize preparation for the meeting. It is likely that the manager will have valuable insight into the existing knowledge base and special characteristics of the new employees. It may be useful for the administrator to review the notes from previous meetings or organize his notes, but these steps should take place after talking with the manager.

68. C: A root cause analysis of inpatient suicides would be most likely to discover problems with the physical environment. Staffing levels, staff orientation, and the availability of information also may contribute to suicide, but the physical environment is much more likely to be involved. Of course, most root cause analyses reveal that there are multiple factors involved in incidents of inpatient suicide.

69. C: One important step towards reducing errors in a system that spans several departments is giving a single person responsibility for overseeing the entire system. Often, the sources of error can only be spotted when a single person examines the system as a whole. It may be impossible for one person to examine in detail the system in every area, but a general supervisor may be able to spot areas in which departments are performing the same functions differently. This sort of inconsistency can lead to errors that may be impossible for department heads to see from their limited perspective.

70. A: In this scenario, the subordinate would be most likely to suggest amendments to the meeting agenda. A content leader is a person who exhibits interest and even mastery of the material with which the group is concerned. When a content leader emerges, administrators should allocate more responsibility to him or her. It should be noted that content leaders are not necessarily easy to work with, because they often become impatient with their colleagues.

71. D: Hospitals include APACHE (acute physiology and chronic health evaluation) III scores in their analysis of infection rate to establish the general likelihood of infection for patients with various conditions. This score is used to determine which patients get certain medicine and to predict the likelihood of morbidity for patients with certain diseases. The inclusion of APACHE III scores on an infection rate analysis might be included to indicate how well the hospital is performing relative to similar institutions.

72. A: As part of the implementation of lean practices, "non-value-add" activities should be minimized or, if possible, eliminated. To classify an activity as "value-add" is to say that its performance increases the value of the product or service. Although it is obvious that a project should maximize value-add activities and minimize non-value-add activities, this is not always possible.

73. C: According to the Joint Commission, the primary cause of wrong-site surgery errors is communication failure. Specifically, these errors are caused by incoherent or incomplete communication between practitioners. Communication factors can be caused by any number of external factors: noisy work environment, lack of a standardized notation system, or bad handwriting to name a few.

74. A: This is a bad strategy because it depends on the vigilance of only one employee. Even the best employees will make mistakes, forget things, or lose their concentration. Important processes should never rely on a single person to repeatedly remember to perform a task. Instead, there should be an automatic alert system that reminds multiple employees that a task needs to be performed.

75. A: One way to create useful alignment in an organization is to base the assessment of each department on the same set of performance dimensions. In lean organizations, alignment is valued because it brings clarity. When all of the departments in an organization are evaluated according to the same dimensions of performance, each employee will be able to assess his own department as well as the other departments. Also, it will be easy for administrators to compare the performances of all the departments.

76. C: In a generic dispensing program, it is not mandatory for the salt form to be the same. Variations in the salt form do not have any measurable effect on the performance of the drug. All of the other answer choices represent essential conditions for generic medications. Many hospitals are able to save money by implementing such programs, but they must be careful to follow the law.

77. C: If administrators are given a list of the variables that predict mortality for patients with a given condition, then they should be able to create a formula for the risk of death for each patient. Such a formula could be used to allocate resources and organize intervention strategies. Also, it could be used to chart the facility's progress in efforts to improve patient outcomes.

78. A: An example of a sentinel event is an unattended and at-risk patient's adverse response to medication. A sentinel event is an adverse occurrence that is not in the normal progression of a patient's illness. The death of a patient from lung cancer would not be considered a sentinel event, for example. However, an adverse drug event is considered a sentinel event, even if the patient is considered to be at risk. Whenever a sentinel event occurs, the healthcare facility should perform a root cause analysis.

79. D: One important driver of customer dissatisfaction in the healthcare industry over the past decade is the improvement of customer care in other service industries. Customers have come to expect a certain standard of care, and as a result are unhappily surprised by their treatment in healthcare facilities. This disparity in treatment is one reason that healthcare administrators have begun to incorporate the strategies and techniques of successful manufacturing and service organizations.

80. D: Patient, clinical, and employee satisfaction are all equally important. That is, they are all targets at which quality improvement efforts should aim. It is common for healthcare facilities to tell the public that patient satisfaction is paramount, to say internally that employee satisfaction is most important, and to act as if clinical satisfaction is the top priority. It is much more productive for an organization to establish concrete performance objectives that will guarantee the satisfaction of all three constituencies.

81. A: The minimum practical lead time for an analytical laboratory is the release constraint test time for the microbiology lab. There is no point to the lead time in the analytical laboratory being any smaller than the release constraint test time for the microbiology lab, because samples can only be processed as quickly as the microbiology lab allows. If the analytical lab reduces lead time below the release constraint test time of the microbiology lab, the resulting difference will simply be slack time.

82. B: A time and materials contract would be most appropriate when remodeling an old wing of a hospital. This type of contract is suitable when the task is difficult to define ahead of time. Remodeling an aging structure can entail hidden costs, such as water or mold damage inside the walls. A time and materials contract states that the contractor will be paid for the overhead, materials, and time required to finish the job.

83. D: In the optimal decision-making process, the most time will be devoted to gathering information. Doing this well depends on effectively framing the issue. Once the issue has been framed, the decision-makers can determine the best sources of information. At the same time, the decision-makers should acknowledge those things that will be impossible to learn or discover. It is important for decision-makers to remain skeptical of their own ability to learn everything of importance about a given issue.

84. D: In lean enterprise, overproduction is the worst type of waste because it contributes to all of the other types. When an organization maintains too much inventory, it becomes inefficient in all areas of operation. Overproduction necessarily wastes time, resources, and effort. One of the fundamental tenets of lean enterprise is the maintenance of an inventory that is no larger than is absolutely necessary.

85. A: Team paralysis is not a common result of rigid adherence to meeting protocol. On the contrary, following the agreed-upon rules for group discussion encourages effective decision-making. Team paralysis is more likely to be caused by ignorance, contentiousness, or an overabundance of options. An effective meeting facilitator will recognize the signs of team paralysis and will intervene to keep the meeting on track.

86. B: A set of key measures that is used to judge progress is known as a dashboard. A dashboard portrays performance as it is happening. It should only include the most essential metrics. Also, the metrics included on a dashboard should be easy to update and monitor because it needs to be accessible at all times. The point of a dashboard is to enable adjustments in real time.

87. C: Volatility in nursing workload is less likely to be reported than other sources of waste because it is less observable. When nurses are busy, they are typically spread out across an entire floor or department. They often have little idea of how busy their colleagues are at any given time. For this reason, it is very difficult to tell when a group of nurses is being deployed inefficiently, or when the workload is particularly volatile. Research has consistently shown that nurses are unable to perceive accurately this volatility unless they are working in close communication.

88. A: An automated pharmacy program that will not fill a prescription unless allergy information has been entered is an example of constraint. Constraints are valuable because they prevent unconscious or involuntary error. In this case, the employees of the pharmacy must answer the allergy question before they can deliver medication. Like a checklist, a constraint places the burden for proper performance on the system rather than the employee.

89. D: The frequency of errors in a particular process would best be displayed in a histogram. Histograms are charts that display the frequencies of various events. It resembles a bar chart, but the bars have varying widths depending on the magnitude of the frequency. A matrix diagram illustrates the relationships between multiple sets of data. A Pareto chart combines a bar graph with a line chart: the bar graph depicts frequencies in descending order, while the line graph illustrates the cumulative total. An affinity diagram illustrates the connections and similarities between items in a set of information.

90. A: One disadvantage of using separate scorecards for financial and customer satisfaction data is that administrators are likely to overvalue the financial information. Even when customer satisfaction is the avowed top priority of an organization, financial concerns nevertheless attract disproportionate attention. For this reason, administrators are encouraged to place all of the important pieces of data on the same scorecard.

91. B: The most common source of the goal statement for a tree diagram is the root cause identified by an interrelationship digraph. Interrelationship digraphs outline all of the factors that influence an issue, and then isolate the one factor that has the most influence. This factor is known as the root cause. On a tree diagram, the root cause will be entered first as the goal statement. Then, the diagram will depict the operations that must be performed to achieve the goal statement.

92. C: One of the consequences of a successful application of the theory of constraints (TOC) is the creation of new constraints. A constraint is the element of a process that restricts efficiency. When TOC is applied successfully, what was once a constraint will be brought up to speed with the rest of the operation. When this happens, other elements of the process may become restrictive to efficiency. In other words, they may become constraints. The TOC model may need to be repeated many times until a system is brought to maximum efficiency.

93. C: Most quality problems in health care are the result of disorganization. In a way, this fact is uplifting, because it suggests that improving quality may not require hiring new employees or purchasing large amounts of new equipment. However, reorganizing processes to achieve superior quality and efficiency can take many years.

94. C: The system limits of a process are typically based on the average and standard deviation of the yield and duration. This means that the system can only be expected to perform within the measured ranges of quantity produced and time of operation. The intention of Six Sigma is to improve the yield and duration and thereby the system limits.

95. A: The administrator is performing a sensitivity analysis. This is a technique for assessing the influences of different inputs on a measurable output. The accuracy of sensitivity analysis is improved when all of the variables are objective and measurable, but it is possible to do a loose analysis by assigning numerical values to subjective variables.

96. B: Over the past three decades, medical knowledge and technology have expanded at an exponential rate. Indeed, the advances made over the past 30 years have moved medicine farther forward than the hundreds of years before them. This sudden and steep rise in the complexity of healthcare has necessitated a high degree of specialization. No one person can be an expert in all of the fields of care. For this reason, effective management is more important than ever.

97. C: A negative binomial distribution could be used to determine the number of blood transfusions that are likely to be performed before an error is made. Negative binomial distributions are effective for indicating how many successful events are likely to occur before a failure. This sort of statistical calculation is useful for monitoring trends in errors.

98. D: An increase in chronic conditions is one consequence of longer life expectancy. As people live longer, they are more likely to develop conditions like dementia, arthritis, and atherosclerosis. As a result, the increase in the incidence of these conditions should not be taken as evidence of poor national health. However, these trends in health should stimulate strategy changes by health care facilities.

99. B: In healthcare, the most common adjustment to the traditional balanced scorecard is the extra emphasis on patient results and customer satisfaction. These elements of performance are important for any business, but they are especially crucial to the success of healthcare facilities. For this reason, the balanced scorecard of a healthcare organization is more likely to make financial and business operations metrics secondary to customer and patient service. The goal of a healthcare organization is to deliver superior service, not to maximize profits.

100. C: The information gathered from customer complaints is considered part of a reactive system. Reactive systems, which depend upon external stimuli, are contrasted with proactive systems, which are initiated by the service provider. Questionnaires, market research, and customer interviews are all proactive. Although a service provider needs to have programs for reaction in place, it is better to elicit market information through proactive means, as this ensures a more accurate and continuous flow of information.

101. D: The "four bads" related to drug-related morbidity are bad drugs, bad patients, bad prescribing, and bad luck. These are the four factors most strongly connected with adverse drug events that lead to death. By addressing these issues, healthcare facilities can reduce medication error and drug-related morbidity.

102. A: The chart will take the form of a T-shaped matrix. This sort of matrix is appropriate for comparing two sets of data to a common third set. The most common arrangement is for two sets of data to run vertically along the left border of the matrix, with the third set running on a horizontal band across the middle. Using the example here, the left border will include values for spending and time, and the horizontal band will name the basic tasks.

103. C: If the load and the mix of a testing laboratory are leveled, the result will be an increase in capacity and/or a reduction in cost. Leveling, also known as smoothing, reduces the volatility of the workload and makes it possible for the lab to process more samples, reduce the costs of operation, or both. This leveling can be accomplished with the implementation of lean practices. The mix of a lab is the composition and diversity of the samples, while the load is the volume of the samples.

104. B: One difference between evidence-based practice and research utilization is that research utilization relies on only one study. Both evidence-based practice and research utilization are objective, data-centered approaches to professional performance, but evidence-based practice is a more holistic incorporation of scientific evidence. Research utilization, on the other hand, is a strategy used by doctors and nurses to solve specific and discrete problems.

105. D: Price information is not one of the basic components of an optimization model. Optimization is a technique for maximizing the utility of limited resources. It requires three elements: an objective function, variable inputs, and constraints. The objective function is a measurable result that needs to be improved. The variable inputs are factors that can be manipulated to affect the objective function. Finally, the constraints are factors that inhibit the effects of the variable inputs.

106. A: At present, the best way to improve the delivery of accurate and useful information would be to create a universal database of patient records. It is not practical to require pharmacists to visit nursing stations regularly, and patients should already have access to their lab reports. Improving the time required for delivery is a positive step, but it will not necessarily improve patient understanding.

107. B: In general, a failure modes and effects analysis (FMEA) should take two steps in each direction. A failure modes and effects analysis is a two-part process: identification of errors or defects (failure modes) and consideration of the consequences (effects analysis). After identifying the causes of error or defect, an FMEA might go on to identify what caused those initial causes. However, proceeding too far down this path can be fruitless. In the same way, evaluating the consequences of the consequences of failure can be productive, but to continue in this direction ultimately generates too much noise to be useful. In some cases, it will be productive to extend FMEA for more than two steps.

108. C: Team members begin to reach consensus on the rules for operation during the stage known as norming. That is, they begin to establish group norms. The four general stages of group behavior are forming (when the group first comes together), storming (when differences are aired and arguments occur), norming, and performing (when the group accomplishes its tasks). Some sociologists include a final recognition stage, in which group members acknowledge the steps that have been taken and resolve to modify their group behavior in the future.

109. D: One characteristic of high-performing groups is a blend of internal focus and external review. In other words, successful groups spend time thinking about their own performance and considering the performance of others. In contrast, groups that are excessively self-interested lose touch with external influences, while groups that are excessively concerned with external elements may become paralyzed. Research suggests that the best groups are by nature optimistic, inquiring, and interested both in their own work and the work of others.

110. A: Framing is the element of decision-making that receives much less time than it deserves. Framing is the process of organizing the question to be decided. It entails listing the possible sources of information and prioritizing the decision-making process. Research suggests that groups tend to spend about five percent of the entire decision-making process on framing when they should spend about 20 percent on it. If a decision is framed well, the subsequent parts of the decision-making process will proceed with relative ease.

111. B: Developing new services is not a goal of quality circles. A quality circle is a small group of employees who perform similar tasks. These employees meet at regular intervals to discuss their jobs and come up with solutions to shared problems. The emphasis of a quality circle is improving existing services, not creating new ones.

112. C: In the most efficient labs, each technician can perform every task, but usually performs only one. When this is the case, the lab has all the benefits of specialization without putting itself at risk of becoming too dependent on a single set of employees. Also, to prevent technicians from becoming bored, many labs will rotate their tasks on a weekly or monthly basis.

113. A: The likelihood that a wheelchair will be available when needed can be calculated with a binomial distribution. A binomial distribution is appropriate for illustrating probabilities when there are two possible events. In this case, the two possible events are that a wheelchair will either be available or not. A healthcare facility could use binomial distributions to determine the likelihood of a wheelchair being available for any given number of wheelchairs. This would be a way to determine the optimal number of wheelchairs for the facility to keep on hand.

114. D: When developing quality standards, the best source of information is external benchmarking data. This data is a map of what is possible in a given field. Healthcare administrators are advised to select an efficient and successful facility and to model their organization after it. One advantage of healthcare is that the nonprofit status of many institutions increases their transparency and cooperation with other organizations.

115. B: Stabilizing total costs is not a primary goal of lean enterprise. Indeed, it is possible that the implementation of lean enterprise practices will raise total costs, at least in the short term. Ultimately, lean enterprise is able to produce greater efficiency, which may translate into lower total costs. The focus of lean enterprise, however, is on the elimination of waste, the reduction of lead times, and (perhaps most importantly) the improvement of quality.

116. C: It is important to use customized benchmarks because external factors may differentiate otherwise similar organizations. For instance, the geographical location of a healthcare facility can have a significant but not obvious effect on statistics. If a facility is located near a lake frequently used for recreation, then there is likely to be an increase in injuries during the warm months when the lake has the most visitors. As much as possible, benchmarks should be customized to provide a true basis for comparison.

117. A: The process in which meeting participants make a list of their priorities and then compile these lists is nominal group technique (NGT). NGT ensures that the opinions of every group member will be taken into account, and that every voice will at least be heard. The other answer choices represent alternate decision-making strategies. Multi-voting is very similar to nominal group technique, except that some participants are allotted more than one vote based on their status within the group.

118. D: Net profit is not one the operational measurements emphasized by the theory of constraints (TOC). However, net profit can be calculated by subtracting operating expense from throughput. In TOC, throughput, inventory, and operating expense are the most important operational measurements. Throughput is the rate at which money is generated, and can be calculated as selling price minus the price of raw materials. Inventory is the amount of investment in salable goods and services. Operating expense is the money spent converting inventory into throughput.

119. B: The best statistical distribution model for examining infrequent infusion equipment errors would be the Poisson distribution. This distribution is best for determining the minimum and maximum number of occurrences of an unlikely event over a specific interval. A binomial distribution describes the probability of two events with known probabilities both happening during the same interval. A normal distribution is arranged like a bell curve, with the most common occurrences in the middle of the range and the least common at either extreme. A multinomial distribution illustrates the probabilities of various results when there are more than two possible results.

120. D: The most common and effective style of checklist for hospital employees prompts a response of "yes" to almost every question. Checklists should serve as external reminders of all the tasks an employee needs to complete, but they should not require a great deal of time or effort. Without checklists, hospital operations may depend on the employees' memories, which are inherently fallible. Checklists should also be easy for supervisors to scan.

121. D: One structural way to avoid groupthink is to have team members submit their comments in writing. Groupthink is an unhealthy tendency towards false consensus. Such a consensus is considered false because it does not represent the true opinions of the group's participants. A group is susceptible to groupthink when its members are ill-informed or insecure in their positions. The leader of a group with this problem may at first be pleased by the ease with which consensus is reached, but will eventually be frustrated by the shallowness of the group's knowledge and the failure to subject ideas to thorough scrutiny. By forcing the group members to submit their comments in writing, the facilitator enables people to express themselves without influence.

122. A: Employee incentive programs should emphasize adherence to established protocols. If performance protocols are clear and appropriate, they should define effective employee behavior. So long as employees abide by these protocols, their performance should be excellent. One characteristic of Six Sigma and other similar management philosophies is the emphasis on processes rather than results. If the processes are performed well, then the results should take care of themselves. If incentives are tied to results, employees may be tempted to cheat or falsify their numbers. In some cases, perfect performance of the task may still result in error. Employees should not be penalized for such events. Instead, this sort of adverse situation should be cause for a reappraisal of the protocols.

123. B: When assessing an emergency room, the best strategy for data collection is continuous sampling. The workload of an emergency room is volatile, so only taking samples from a limited interval can create a distorted statistical picture. Instead, samples should be collected at regular and frequent intervals, so that the peaks and valleys of the workload are represented in the data.

124. C: A broad collection of health-care providers, support personnel, and private contractors is not one of the four elements of a health service microsystem. A health service microsystem is a small, self-sufficient group of front-line practitioners. Most people in the United States receive their care from a health service microsystem. Contrary to a broad collection, a health service microsystem includes a defined set of service providers.

125. C: One advantage of a voluntary error reporting system over a mandatory reporting system is that voluntary systems elicit more reports from front-line practitioners. Research has consistently shown that doctors and nurses who work directly with patients are more likely to report errors when there is a voluntary system in place. Error reporting is a crucial area in quality improvement. An effective system is necessary for the acquisition of accurate data. At present, there is no standardized error-reporting system in healthcare, although there are several common models.

126. A: The main difference between the Taguchi model of service provision and the traditional model is that the Taguchi model identifies waste any time a process deviates from its target. In the traditional model, on the other hand, a process is considered optimal so long as it falls within a broad set of specifications. The Taguchi model brings a sense of perfectionism to service provision. It establishes ideal conditions, and then notes any areas in which the operation falls short. For this reason, it is better at informing quality improvement efforts.

127. D: After making a list of the factors that influence this issue, the team will draw relationship arrows between the factors. An interrelationship digraph, also known as a relations diagram, illustrates the causal connections between the factors associated with a particular issue. The factors are written down, and then arrows are drawn from the influencing factor to the factor being influenced. It is possible for two factors to influence one another. Whichever factor has the most outgoing arrows is identified as the root driver, while the factor with the most incoming arrows is identified as the essential outcome.

128. D: One common result of creating a fast track for urgent samples is that the portion of samples placed in the fast track will steadily increase. Typically, lab managers establish basic guidelines for which samples belong in the fast track, but as time passes, these standards are relaxed and a greater number of samples are placed on the accelerated track. Eventually, the fast track has queues similar to those that inspired its creation in the first place. As a result, it is simply better to speed up the processing of all samples than it is to create a special fast track.

129. A: A Kano diagram is appropriate for categorizing the needs of customers. In a classic Kano diagram (also known as a Kano model) the qualities of a product are broken down into five categories: attractive (pleasant but not necessary), one-dimensional (valued when fulfilled, disappointing when unfulfilled), must-be (assumed to be present, deal-breaking when unfulfilled), indifferent (neither positive nor negative), and reverse (valuable to some customers, unimportant to others).

130. B: The most important characteristic of the controls in a case-control study is that they are identical to the cases in every respect except for the presence of the targeted condition. Otherwise, there are too many variables that could skew the results of the study. It is not necessary for the controls to be drawn from a random pool of patients. On the contrary, researchers will frequently need to exercise extreme care in the selection of controls. Many studies do not require frequent observation, and very few require the controls to be literate.

131. A: When a hospital administration decides on strategy, this information should be shared with employees, patients, and the community. Indeed, a hospital's strategic decisions should be shared with any interested parties. However, there are occasional situations in which the facility will need to keep information confidential. For instance, there may be legal reasons for failing to disclose a planned merger with another healthcare provider. However, a hospital will benefit from transparency more often than not. Research suggests that transparent organizations win more buy-in from employees, and more trust from patients. In addition, openness about strategy can elicit helpful criticism.

132. C: Applying the central limit theorem means that the administrator will assume that a sample is representative of the department as a whole. The central limit theorem asserts that when a sufficiently large sample is taken, its characteristics can be expected to represent the entire population. For this theorem to hold, the sampling technique must be appropriate to the subject.

133. B: One common problem in labs with low turnover is narrow specialization by technicians. When technicians are unable to fulfill multiple duties within a laboratory, it becomes more difficult for the lab to operate at peak efficiency. The best model is for technicians to specialize in one area but be capable of performing several, if not all, of the other tasks.

134. B: Frequent benchmarking is important in lean service because it prevents an organization from failing to react to external changes. Lean service providers are in constant contact with the outside world through their customers, but in some cases, they may be slow to acknowledge changes in the market. Benchmarking highlights any important external factors and brings them to the attention of management.

135. A: Root cause analyses most often reveal that mistakes are the result of a series of small errors. Moreover, mistakes and system failures are likely to be predicated on a series of small and often latent errors. This is one reason why it is impossible for front-line practitioners to eradicate errors through diligence and great effort. It is instead necessary for administrators and quality improvement managers to examine processes in their totality and eliminate sources of error.

136. A: The strongest basis for practice is systematic reviews of randomized clinical trials. These reviews provide the most objective and advanced medical knowledge. The other three answer choices represent solid but fallible sources of information. In particular, practitioners should be skeptical about the views of opinion leaders unless these views are clearly based on established clinical research.

137. D: Research suggests that people make fewer errors when they work in a team. There are a few reasons for this. First, the desire to demonstrate competency in front of peers encourages people to attend more fully to their tasks. Also, the members of a group are able to correct one another. People do tend to make more errors when they work creatively, although these errors often lead to insight and innovation. Multi-tasking, however, increases the likelihood of error without providing any benefit. Research consistently shows that people who perform more than one task at the same time are less successful at each of the tasks.

138. C: A brief analysis of interventions for stroke is likely to be relatively unhelpful because research has yet to discover an effective standard treatment. Several treatments may be effective in certain circumstances. A large percentage of stroke victims die almost immediately, and many are elderly and already suffering from other ailments, both of which are factors that increase the difficulty of effective intervention analysis.

139. D: Hospitals pay special attention to blood transfusions because they are complicated and dangerous. Even though transfusions are performed frequently, they are still prone to occasional errors. These errors can be injurious and even fatal. Not all transfusion errors will be detected, however. Hospitals should establish clear protocols with significant rechecking for blood transfusions.

140. D: The main difference between a dashboard and a scorecard is that a scorecard describes past performance, while a dashboard depicts performance in real time. Indeed, a dashboard is so-called because it is analogous to the dashboard of a car, which delivers current metrics. Dashboards are better for making quick adjustments, whereas scorecards are better at providing a comprehensive, clear-eyed view of performance over the recent past.

Practice Test #2

1. The type of power that a staff nurse obtains by closely affiliating with the unit supervisor is:

    a. connective.
    b. coercive.
    c. legitimate.
    d. referent.

2. When building a team, a key strategy must include:

    a. demonstrating authority.
    b. being consistently positive.
    c. managing emotions/feelings.
    d. exhibiting self-confidence.

3. Rate-based measures are expressed as:

    a. precise numbers.
    b. proportions/ratios.
    c. range of numbers.
    d. virtual numbers.

4. If a reimbursement method is going to change, and a date (6 months in the future) and a grace period (an additional 3 months) have been set for implementation, the best time to begin to implement the change is:

    a. immediately.
    b. in 4 months (before implementation).
    c. in 6 months (at implementation).
    d. before end of the grace period.

5. In survey design, "operational definition" refers to terms:

    a. used to provide directions.
    b. related to surgical procedures.
    c. that include medical jargon.
    d. understood by researchers and participants.

6. Material safety data sheets (MDSSs) must be available:

    a. on file in Administration.
    b. in each department.
    c. upon request.
    d. at locations of hazardous materials.

7. When carrying out process improvement projects, an affinity diagram is used to:

    a. outline cause and effect.
    b. organize and prioritize ideas.
    c. outline process steps.
    d. establish a timeline.

8. Which of the following has been shown to consistently reduce hospital-associated adverse events?

    a. Punitive measures.
    b. Interdisciplinary teams.
    c. Increased nurse-to-patient ratio.
    d. Early discharge.

9. The type of leadership that is most likely to stifle creative problem-solving is:

    a. bureaucratic.
    b. charismatic.
    c. democratic.
    d. laissez-faire.

10. According to the Change Theory (Lewin, Schein), the first stage, motivation to change (unfreezing), may be characterized by:

    a. overriding of defensive actions.
    b. change in perceptions of self and relationships.
    c. identification of needed changes.
    d. survival anxiety and learning anxiety.

11. Emergency planning should begin with:

    a. hazard vulnerability analysis.
    b. survey of other institutions' policies.
    c. review of past emergencies.
    d. cost assessment.

12. The type of database that is generally utilized to track such things as inventory and purchases is a(n):

    a. relational database.
    b. operational database.
    c. hierarchical database.
    d. real-time database.

13. If the purpose of a project is to develop a new emergency preparedness plan, the document that is provided at the end of the project would be categorized as a:

    a. plan.
    b. report.
    c. deliverable.
    d. product.

14. If utilizing the Lean-Six Sigma approach to performance improvement, the primary focus should be on:

    a. execution of project by project.
    b. strategic goals.
    c. cost-effectiveness.
    d. identification of errors.

15. If the organization's overall staff turnover rate exceeds the benchmark (<6%) set by the organization, the next step should be to:

    a. analyze the rate by job class.
    b. survey all staff regarding job satisfaction.
    c. develop a strategy for retention.
    d. carry out a salary comparison study.

16. Which of the following characteristics suggests that a team is likely to be ineffective?

    a. Leadership shifts periodically.
    b. Conflicts are discussed openly.
    c. Constructive criticism is freely given.
    d. Two members dominate team meetings.

17. The measures presented in a balanced scorecard should be based on the organization's:

    a. mission, vision, goals, and objectives.
    b. cost-effectiveness analysis.
    c. accreditation requirements.
    d. patient satisfaction surveys.

18. Which of the following tools may be used to best develop and manage a timeline for a quality improvement project?

    a. Story board.
    b. Task list.
    c. GANTT chart.
    d. Affinity diagram.

19. If one unit in the hospital that has a far lower rate of hospital-associated infections than similar units is used as a performance indicator for comparison, this is an example of:

    a. functional benchmarking.
    b. internal benchmarking.
    c. generic benchmarking.
    d. competitive benchmarking.

20. When using a run chart with more than 21 data points to analyze data, 7 or more consecutive data points in ascending order would be classified as a(n):

    a. run.
    b. cycle.
    c. astronomical value.
    d. trend.

21. Third party payers, such as insurance companies, are most likely to assess the quality of patient care based on:

    a. access to care.
    b. patient outcomes.
    c. cost-effectiveness.
    d. technical performance.

22. CMS contracts with nongovernmental quality improvement organizations (QIOs), whose job is to monitor patient care by:

    a. onsite interviews and observations.

    b. retrospective review of patient records.

    c. conducting patient satisfaction surveys.

    d. auditing coding and billing procedures.

23. In a scattergram, if the data begin to form a straight-line pattern, this is evidence that:

    a. there is a correlation between the two variables.

    b. there is no correlation between the two variables. ·

    c. no conclusion can be reached regarding correlation.

    d. data were incorrectly plotted.

24. Based on HHS guidelines for pandemic planning, if 500,000 people in the local population fall ill, what number is likely to seek outpatient medical care?

    a. 50,000.

    b. 100,000.

    c. 250,000.

    d. 400,000.

25. What percentage of data points normally fall within one standard deviation of the mean?

    a. 33%.

    b. 68%.

    c. 95%.

    d. 99%.

26. What type of error in measurement may occur if the participant reacts to the interviewer's lack of friendliness?

    a. Response set bias.

    b. Situational contamination.

    c. Transitory personal factor.

    d. Administrative variation.

27. The primary goal of the continuum of care is to provide healthcare:

    a. throughout a patient's life.

    b. that is cost effective.

    c. without adverse effects.

    d. to the point of optimal health.

28. When analyzing variability, the semi-interquartile range (SIQR) uses:

    a. 100% of data.

    b. 75% of data.

    c. 50% of data.

    d. 25% of data.

29. If, as part of a research project, an analysis of the null hypothesis results in a p-value of 0.001, this suggests that:

    a. the null hypothesis is wrong.
    b. the null hypothesis is correct.
    c. the null hypothesis may or may not be correct.
    d. the null hypothesis cannot be evaluated.

30. According to force field analysis (Lewin), the two forces that must be considered for change include:

    a. costs and benefits.
    b. time and effort.
    c. staff and administration.
    d. driving and restraining.

31. If the process improvement team leader assigns a team facilitator, that individual's role is to:

    a. schedule meetings.
    b. manage conflicts and group dynamics.
    c. record information.
    d. coordinate data collection.

32. If the hospital has established a goal of reducing pressure sores by establishing and monitoring set time periods for turning patients, what type of health promotion and preventative effort does this represent?

    a. Primary.
    b. Secondary.
    c. Tertiary.
    d. Quaternary.

33. Which of the following provides quality indicators, such as Prevention Quality Indicators and Patient Safety Indicators?

    a. AHRQ.
    b. TJC.
    c. IHI.
    d. NCQA.

34. According to the National Quality Forum (NQF), if a patient dies from a fall while hospitalized, this type of serious reportable event (SRE) would be reported as a(n):

    a. care management event.
    b. environmental event.
    c. criminal event.
    d. patient protection event.

35. According to the IHI, the four criteria for Always Events are (1) important, (2) evidence-based, (3) measurable, and (4):

    a. beneficial.
    b. functional.
    c. ongoing/continuous.
    d. affordable/sustainable.

36. When conducting education or training programs for adults, it's important to remember that, according to the Theory of Andragogy (Knowles), adult learners tend to be:

    a. enlightened.
    b. self-directed.
    c. aggressive.
    d. defensive.

37. Which of the following immunizations does the CDC currently recommend for all healthcare workers who cannot demonstrate immunity?

    a. Hepatitis B.
    b. Pneumococcal.
    c. Herpes zoster (shingles).
    d. Meningococcal.

38. The primary problem with assessing performance through direct observation is:

    a. it is time intensive.
    b. assessment is subjective.
    c. performance may change under observation.
    d. difficulty establishing criteria.

39. Preadmission services should base admission criteria on:

    a. age and gender.
    b. insurance coverage.
    c. possible diagnosis.
    d. prognosis.

40. How many individuals usually form a quality circle?

    a. 1 to 2.
    b. 3 to 4.
    c. 5 to 10.
    d. 10 to 15.

41. If a sample is obtained by enrolling all patients who come to an outpatient clinic until the target number of participants is reached, the type of sampling utilized is:

    a. convenience sampling.
    b. purposive sampling.
    c. quota sampling.
    d. cluster sampling.

42. If, for clinical research regarding patient concerns, staff nurses in multiple departments will be provided questionnaires to administer to patients, the biggest concern regarding this method of data collection is likely:

    a. time factors.
    b. consistency.
    c. cost.
    d. sample size

43. Which of the following ultimately defines organizational quality?

a. Senior administration.
b. Regulatory agency.
c. Staff members.
d. Customers.

44. When designing educational activities, the first step is to determine the:

a. costs.
b. time needed.
c. purpose.
d. expected outcomes.

45. When utilizing the FOCUS methodology for quality improvement, the U stands for:

a. utilization of resources.
b. uncover the reasons for the problem.
c. undergo organizational self-assessment.
d. unify standards or care.

46. When planning a staff meeting to discuss quality improvement initiatives, the CPHQ should first:

a. develop the agenda.
b. send out meeting announcements.
c. post meeting time and location.
d. plan a free-form discussion.

47. The primary disadvantage of mailed surveys is:

a. they are prohibitively expensive.
b. return times vary widely.
c. the return rate is low.
d. participants cannot ask questions.

48. When facilitating quality improvement, the biggest barrier to implementation of changes is usually:

a. administration.
b. staff resistance.
c. cost constraints.
d. time constraints.

49. As part of performance improvement, the Ishikawa (fishbone) diagram may be used to help to identify:

a. gaps in performance.
b. relationships between 2 variables.
c. steps in a process.
d. root causes.

50. When making a process map as part of needs assessment, the CPHQ must map the process as:

    a. it actually takes place.
    b. it should take place.
    c. it will take place.
    d. people report it takes place.

51. If, when monitoring a quality improvement project, the CPHQ notes that all deliverables have been consistently behind schedule for the past 8 weeks, the best initial approach is to:

    a. speed up the process.
    b. identify weak links.
    c. adjust the timeline.
    d. provide incentives.

52. A complete history and physical examination should be completed on an inpatient with no recent history of care within:

    a. 6 hours.
    b. 12 hours.
    c. 18 hours.
    d. 24 hours.

53. The Plan-Do-Check-Act (PDCA) (Shewhart cycle) method of continuous quality improvement is best suited for:

    a. organization-wide problems.
    b. specific problems.
    c. interdisciplinary problems.
    d. community-wide problems.

54. If a "never event" occurs, the initial response should be to:

    a. identify culpable staff members.
    b. assume no responsibility.
    c. accept liability.
    d. conduct a root-cause analysis.

55. If a hospital is interested in applying for the Magnet Recognition Program® through the ANCC, the first step is to:

    a. conduct a gap analysis.
    b. conduct a need assessment.
    c. consult an advisor.
    d. form a magnet team.

56. An innovation adopter who doesn't propose innovations but is willing to readily adopt them when proposed by others would be categorized as:

    a. late majority.
    b. early adopter.
    c. early majority.
    d. laggard.

57. Which of the following accreditation organizations for hospitals, critical access hospitals, and ancillary services (home health agency, hospice) provides a number of certificates, including Managing Infection Risk and Primary Stroke Center?

    a. CARF.
    b. DNV GL.
    c. TJC.
    d. AAAHC.

58. What is the primary purpose of rapid cycle testing?

    a. Reduce time needed for implementation.
    b. Eliminate the need for ongoing evaluation.
    c. Justify a process improvement process.
    d. Reduce the costs of implementation.

59. Which ISO standard covers quality management and promotes a process approach utilizing the PDCA cycle?

    a. ISO 6000.
    b. ISO 7000.
    c. ISO 8000.
    d. ISO 9000.

60. What is the appropriate initial response if the hospital has received an onsite OSHA inspection because of a complaint filed by a worker about safety concerns?

    a. Try to ascertain the name of the worker.
    b. Take steps to remedy the safety concern.
    c. Call a staff meeting to discuss safety concerns.
    d. File a counterclaim citing the hospital's safety record.

61. What is the first step that must be carried out for an organization utilizing the Baldridge Excellence Framework to promote excellence?

    a. Complete a cost assessment.
    b. Carry out a needs assessment.
    c. Create an organization profile.
    d. Assess staff commitment.

62. When should preparation for Joint Commission accreditation inspections be carried out?

    a. On a continuous basis.
    b. Annually.
    c. Six months prior to the inspection.
    d. Three months prior to the inspection.

63. If an outbreak of *Clostridium difficile* has occurred resulting in multiple cases of severe diarrhea in hospitalized patients and staff members on one unit, the initial infection control efforts should be aimed at:

    a. isolating patients with the infection.
    b. closing the unit for disinfection.
    c. penalizing staff members.
    d. hand washing procedures.

64. If a patient satisfaction survey covers topics clearly related to issues of patient satisfaction, the type of validity the survey has is:

    a. criterion validity.
    b. discriminant validity.
    c. content validity.
    d. convergent validity.

65. According to the Pyramid of Evidence (Haynes), AKA the 5 S's (Studies, Syntheses, Synopses, Summaries, and Systems), which of the following would be categorized under Syntheses?

    a. Detailed description of research project.
    b. Meta-analyses.
    c. Case studies.
    d. Concept analysis.

66. To ensure that new hires are correctly licensed and credentialed, it is necessary to:

    a. ask the individual for detailed information.
    b. require presentation of licenses and credentials.
    c. contact previous employers.
    d. carry out a primary source verification.

67. A process improvement team comprised only of members from one department or service area is categorized as a:

    a. functional team.
    b. blitz team.
    c. cross-functional team.
    d. self-directed team.

68. Which of the following narrative documentations in EHRs is most appropriate?

    a. "Patient complaining constantly about care."
    b. "Patient states that he has not received assistance with bathing or dental care."
    c. "Patient wants more personal care."
    d. "Patient is very unhappy with care being received."

69. What are the 4 core criteria for credentialing and privileging?

    a. Licensure, performance ability, recommendation, necessity.
    b. Education, licensure, necessity, and recommendation.
    c. Licensure, education, competence, performance ability.
    d. Recommendation, education, licensure, experience.

70. Which of the following is a method used to measure instrument reliability?

    a. Internal consistency measures.
    b. Scale reliability coefficient.
    c. Instrumental calculation.
    d. Test-retest reliability coefficient.

71. **What is the most important element of a disaster/emergency preparedness plan?**

    a. Readily available information and practice drills.
    b. Transfer protocols.
    c. Triage.
    d. Chain of command.

72. **Medical orders for behavioral restraints for those ages 9 through 17 are time-limited to:**

    a. 8 hours.
    b. 6 hours.
    c. 4 hours.
    d. 2 hours.

73. **If data include patients' blood pressures, these data are categorized as:**

    a. nominal.
    b. continuous.
    c. ordinal.
    d. discrete.

74. **Principles of high-reliability organizations include:**

    a. staff loyalty to the organization.
    b. constant concern with cost-effectiveness.
    c. constant concern regarding failure.
    d. routine recognition and rewards for quality service.

75. **When evaluating Internet sources as part of literature review and research, the two most important criteria are:**

    a. content and credibility.
    b. copyright and context.
    c. continuity and compatibility.
    d. citation and connectivity.

76. **Which of the following is the abstract database of the National Library of Medicine?**

    a. *CINAHL*.
    b. *OVID*.
    c. *EBSCO*.
    d. *PubMed*.

77. **If a hospital is part of a provider network but contracts with providers (such as anesthesiologists) who are not in the plan's network, resulting in multiple complaints of "surprise bills," the hospital should:**

    a. leave the matter to legal counsel.
    b. notify patient's in advance of estimated costs.
    c. utilize only in-network providers.
    d. ignore complaints as part of doing business.

78. If the data set includes 68, 82, 86, 89, 90, 90, 91, 91, 92, 92 and 94, the median value is:

    a. 89
    b. 89.5
    c. 90
    d. 90.5

79. If the CPHQ has determined that the hospital can better improve trauma care with the data provided by a trauma registry, the next step is to develop the:

    a. protocol for case finding.
    b. protocol for submission of data.
    c. reporting schedule.
    d. case definition.

80. What is the primary purpose of the Healthcare Effective Data and Information Set (HEDIS) tool?

    a. Measure performance.
    b. Reduce costs.
    c. Set performance goals.
    d. Assess best practices.

81. Before instituting organization-wide utilization of SBAR for hand-offs and transitions of care, the CPHQ should initially:

    a. survey the staff.
    b. provide guidelines and training.
    c. mandate a date for implementation.
    d. advise staff to research SBAR.

82. What four types of quality measures are pay-for-performance programs usually based on?

    a. Costs, outcomes, timeliness, and best practices.
    b. Performance, costs, outcomes, and patient experience.
    c. Performance, outcomes, patient experience, and structure/technology.
    d. Patient experience, outcomes, costs, and timeliness.

83. According to the general systems theory, which of the following would be classified as an output?

    a. Praise.
    b. Facts.
    c. Lived experience.
    d. Changed behavior.

84. A team is best described as:

    a. Leaders and followers engaged in some activity.
    b. Individuals with common goals.
    c. Individuals assembled together with a mutual interest.
    d. Individuals working together to carry out a specific activity.

85. According to Westrum's phases of safety culture, an organization that indicates a concern for safety and takes action when an accident occurs to prevent a recurrence is in what phase?

    a. Calculative.
    b. Pathological.
    c. Reactive.
    d. Generative.

86. After selecting a number of possible vendors for a complex upgrade of equipment and services, the next step is to develop a:

    a. business plan.
    b. request for proposal.
    c. request for quotation.
    d. budget allowance.

87. Under the Joint Commission's policies, which of the following is a reviewable sentinel event for hospitals?

    a. Suicide within 72 hours of discharge.
    b. Death of a preterm infant.
    c. Theft of personal belongings.
    d. Assault resulting in contusions.

88. Which of the following reportable diseases requires a mandatory written report?

    a. Varicella (chicken pox).
    b. Influenza.
    c. Pertussis.
    d. Gonorrhea.

89. A patient safety event that reaches the patient in some manner but does not result in harm to the patient is categorized as:

    a. adverse event.
    b. close call.
    c. no-harm event.
    d. hazardous condition.

90. Which nursing care delivery system is most economical but fragments care?

    a. Functional care.
    b. Primary care.
    c. Team nursing.
    d. Total care.

91. Which of the following outlines systematic procedures based on a patient's treatment response, such as for asthma care?

    a. Protocol.
    b. Clinical pathway.
    c. Algorithm.
    d. Guideline.

92. When assessing quality performance, the degree to which an intervention accomplishes desired outcomes refers to its:

    a. efficiency.
    b. appropriateness.
    c. effectiveness.
    d. efficacy.

93. When assessing the core measure related to use of high-risk medications in the elderly, most data will likely be obtained from:

    a. patient interviews.
    b. EHRs.
    c. physician surveys.
    d. patient surveys.

94. The primary component of a life safety management program is:

    a. fire prevention plan.
    b. information backup plan.
    c. utilities management.
    d. staffing protocols.

95. If hospital administration mandates a change in skill mix to decrease the number of registered nurses in order to save costs and cope with a nursing shortage, the first step should be to:

    a. determine the tasks that must be done by RNs.
    b. calculate the reduction in RNs needed to meet target cost reduction.
    c. determine the tasks that can be done by non-RNs.
    d. conduct a survey of wages for different types of staff.

96. If a hospital has instituted a just culture to encourage staff to report incidents and unsafe practices, a nurse who misread a medication order and administered an incorrect dosage to a patient should be:

    a. placed on probation.
    b. provided a coach and further training.
    c. fired for incompetence.
    d. consoled and supported.

97. Which of the following poses a potential risk of infant/child abduction?

    a. Fire alarms disengage door locks.
    b. Mothers and infants have identical ID bands.
    c. Employees wear ID badges with color photos.
    d. There is one public entry to the nursery area.

98. What is the primary advantage of "smart pumps" over standard infusion pumps?

    a. Ease of operation.
    b. Decreased cost of maintenance.
    c. Error prevention.
    d. Flexibility.

99. If a power outage delayed surgeries when the backup power system failed, this would be classified as a:

    a. common cause variation.
    b. special cause variation.
    c. random variation.
    d. direct variation.

100. When establishing hospital standard measures, what is an appropriate benchmark for admitting patients for observation who actually meet criteria for inpatient admission?

    a. <3%.
    b. <2%.
    c. <1%.
    d. 0%.

101. When preparing data for display, which of the following may be distracting to the viewer?

    a. Font size 14 is used for text and size 16 for headings.
    b. Text is against a bright yellow background.
    c. The Verdana font is used for text.
    d. Highlighted text is underlined.

102. Once an evidence-based change has been implemented, the next critical element is to:

    a. measure outcomes.
    b. survey staff.
    c. assess costs.
    d. punish non-compliance.

103. According to Hospital Compare, the most common overall rating for hospitals is:

    a. 1 star.
    b. 2 stars.
    c. 3 stars.
    d. 4 stars.

104. If one of the hospital's strategic goals is to enhance the organization's clinical capabilities, which of the following improvement projects would have priority?

    a. Expanding the emergency department to become a trauma center.
    b. Investing in updated technology, including digital tools for patients.
    c. Providing educational programs for community members.
    d. Entering partnerships with health systems and provider organizations.

105. When using the PICOT format to research best practices, the P represents:

    a. perception.
    b. phenomenon.
    c. parameter.
    d. patient/population.

106. If present-on-admission indicators for diagnoses have been frequently overlooked for patients because of inadequate data collection and evaluation, the most likely impact for the organization is:

    a. negligible impact.
    b. misclassification as complications.
    c. inadequate patient care.
    d. decreased patient satisfaction.

107. If utilizing the CRAF method to record minutes of meetings of the process improvement team, CRAF stands for:

    a. control, report, activities, and feedback.
    b. consensus, results, alternatives, and future plans.
    c. conclusions, recommendations, actions, and follow-up.
    d. conditions, resolutions, advice, and flow chart.

108. To comply with OSHA regulations, a healthcare worker exposed to HIV through a needlestick must be monitored after exposure for at least:

    a. 12 months.
    b. 8 months.
    c. 6 months.
    d. 3 months.

109. The purpose of a data-flow diagram is to show how:

    a. research processes were carried out.
    b. data flow into a system and from one process to another.
    c. reports are disseminated throughout an organization.
    d. the EHR connects to pharmacy and other departments.

110. The degree to which the user of data is able to understand the rationale behind the date and the outcomes refers to the data's:

    a. interpretability.
    b. reliability.
    c. validity.
    d. stability.

111. Considering safety concerns, which of the following occurring in a community may most impact the security management of a hospital?

    a. Recent string of bank robberies.
    b. Increasing immigrant population.
    c. Increased rates of heroin addiction.
    d. Opening of a new federal prison.

112. Juran's "quality trilogy" comprises quality planning, quality improvement, and quality:

    a. evaluation.
    b. product.
    c. outcomes.
    d. control.

113. If a patient gives permission for a staff person to accompany her throughout a visit and take notes of the experience, this is an example of:

a. patient shadowing.
b. walk-through.
c. process review.
d. gap analysis.

114. Which of the following poses an increased risk of infection?

a. Windows that won't open.
b. Frayed cords on equipment.
c. Water-stained ceiling tiles.
d. Pharmacy-filled medication carts.

115. With the RACE method of dealing with a fire, the C stands for:

a. Conduct evacuation.
b. Confine fires.
c. Coordinate activities.
d. Contact fire department.

116. To determine whether an applicant requesting clinical privileges has settled malpractice claims, the organization must:

a. ask the applicant.
b. query the appropriate state medical board.
c. query the National Practitioner Data Bank.
d. query previous employers.

117. If the Joint Commission grants contingent accreditation, the organization is generally subject to a follow-up survey in:

a. 12 months.
b. 6 months.
c. 3 months.
d. 30 days.

118. Which of the following steps takes place during the initiation phase of the process improvement cycle?

a. Estimate timeline for activities.
b. Begin training program.
c. Create mission and vision statements.
d. Develop criteria for standards.

119. In a PERT (Program Evaluation and Review Technique) chart, parallel activities:

a. occur at the same time.
b. involve the same activity.
c. require the same amount of time.
d. are carried out by the same individual(s).

120. If implementing more streamlined procedures results in a lighter workload but elimination of some staff positions, the likely response to remaining staff will be:

    a. acceptance.
    b. anxiety.
    c. enthusiasm.
    d. disinterest.

121. What is the first step in change management?

    a. Acknowledge losses.
    b. Provide information.
    c. Request input and feedback.
    d. Identify losses.

122. The four basic elements of malpractice include (1) duty to use due care, (2) breach of duty, (3) damages, and (4):

    a. causation.
    b. intent.
    c. liability.
    d. conspiracy.

123. Before construction begins on a renovation project, what assessment(s) should be completed?

    a. Risk management.
    b. Quality measures.
    c. Life safety and infection control.
    d. Medical equipment and materials.

124. Under tort law, a nurse who tells an uncooperative patient that he is being ridiculous and threatens to carry out a treatment on the patient against the patient's will may be charged with:

    a. battery.
    b. assault.
    c. false imprisonment.
    d. defamation of character.

125. In the case of malpractice, peer review information (such as records of discussions and decisions) is:

    a. discoverable.
    b. privileged.
    c. protected.
    d. liable.

126. In human factor engineering, forcing function refers to:

    a. using checklists and standardized equipment/processes.
    b. identifying workarounds that staff members have developed.
    c. anticipating problems in the workplace.
    d. requiring a specific step before another step can be performed.

127. According to Havelock's (1973) Six Phases of Planned Change, the first phase involves:

    a. building relationship with the system.
    b. diagnosing problems.
    c. obtaining necessary resources.
    d. selecting a solution.

128. If a nurse promises to check on a patient every hour and follows through on the promise, the nurse is exhibiting adherence to the ethical principle of:

    a. veracity.
    b. fidelity.
    c. advocacy.
    d. beneficence.

129. The purpose of selecting a trigger for each measure of performance is to indicate when:

    a. to begin the process improvement process.
    b. a process improvement project is completed.
    c. the analytical process is completed.
    d. further analysis needs to be carried out.

130. For staffing purposes, a staff nurse who works 20 hours a week throughout the year would be considered:

    a. 2.0 FTEs.
    b. 1.0 FTE.
    c. 0.5 FTE.
    d. 0.2 FTE.

131. The first stage of strategic planning involves:

    a. external and internal environment assessment.
    b. review of mission, goals, and objectives.
    c. identifying a list of possible strategies.
    d. conducting a cost-effectiveness analysis.

132. If a team leader states, "I am worried about nurse X's anger and hostility and wonder how I can help to reduce tension," the communication pattern the team member is using is:

    a. placation.
    b. congruence.
    c. irrelevance.
    d. blame.

133. When dealing with conflict in a team, which of the following would be classified as an unconscious reactive response?

    a. Showing respect.
    b. Accepting accountability.
    c. Expressing feelings.
    d. Blaming others.

134. The most essential step in supply management is:

    a. control of inventory.
    b. establishing relationships with suppliers.
    c. effective purchasing.
    d. administrative oversight.

135. The primary purpose of workflow analysis of processes is to:

    a. determine cost-effectiveness.
    b. identify bottlenecks.
    c. provide a timeline.
    d. identify key stakeholders.

136. If a security breach involving a patient's EHR occurred when a nurse logged in to the EHR and then left the computer without logging out and a visitor read information on the computer screen, the best solution is to:

    a. add an automatic log-off feature.
    b. take punitive actions against the nurse.
    c. post signs reminding users to log out.
    d. verbally remind staff to log out.

137. The type of implementation in which a complete new system goes live at the same time across an organization, such as a switch from paper documentation to an EHR, is referred to as a:

    a. phased/rollout implementation.
    b. pilot implementation.
    c. parallel implementation.
    d. big bang implementation.

138. If information from patient EHRs has been shared with unauthorized individuals, the best approach to identifying how the breach occurred is to:

    a. interview staff members.
    b. carry out audit trails.
    c. ask for anonymous reports.
    d. provide rewards for information.

139. When gathering data and assessing risks as part of the risk management team, the best approach is to use:

    a. qualitative measures.
    b. quantitative measures.
    c. multiple measures.
    d. observations.

140. Which type(s) of plans for change in condition should be included in patients' discharge care plans?

    a. expected changes.
    b. unexpected changes.
    c. expected and unexpected changes.
    d. emergent changes.

Answer Key and Explanations for Test #2

1. D: The type of power that a staff nurse obtains by closely affiliating with the unit supervisor is referent power. That is, others may feel that the personal or professional connection that exists might allow the person to influence supervisorial decisions. The degree of referent power that the nurse has is a direct reflection of the degree of respect (or fear) that the staff members hold for the supervisor. Referent power may be respected or resented.

2. C: When building a team, a key strategy must include managing emotions/feelings. While responding to negative emotions (anger, frustration, anxiety) can adversely affect team members and result in intimidation, lack of confidence, and resentment, suppressing emotions can also have negative effects on the individual (withdrawal, stress, fear, lack of motivation), which can in turn affect other team members. Emotions and feelings should be routinely acknowledged and discussed so they don't build up and overwhelm team members.

3. B: Rate-based measures are expressed as proportions or ratios. A ratio compares occurrences (such as cases of pneumonia) to a related phenomenon or condition (total cases of influenza). Ratio basically looks at an entire population (as defined by the research) and determines how many within that population have a specific condition/attribute. Ratios are also often used to compare an organization's performance with benchmarks and to show the relationship between data, such as for nurse-patient ratios.

4. A: If a reimbursement method is going to change and a date (6 months in the future) and a grace period (an additional 3 months) have been set for implementation, the best time to begin to implement the change is immediately. Implementation may require programming, staff training, data collection, and other activities, so preparation should begin when notice is received so that the organization is ready at the time of implementation.

5. D: In survey design, "operational definition" refers to terms understood by both researchers and participants. Medical jargon, vocabulary, and terminology that the average person may not understand should be avoided in surveys as they may intimidate the participant and discourage participation. Additionally, participants may misunderstand questions and, therefore, answer incorrectly. Most consumer medical information should be written at a 4th to 6th grade level, and this is also appropriate for many consumer surveys.

6. D: Material safety data sheet (MDSSs) must be available at locations of hazardous materials. The MDSS should outline safety procedures and any potential hazards. MDSS must identify the chemicals, explain their characteristics (such as boiling point), outline fire/explosion hazards and any reactivity as well as health hazards. Personal protective equipment needed for handling must be outlined and any special precaution, such as for handling, transportation, or storage.

7. B: When carrying out process improvement projects, an affinity diagram is used to organize and prioritize ideas garnered during brainstorming. Adhesive notes, such as Post-it® notes, are often utilized for affinity diagrams. Based on the results of brainstorming, a number of different categories are generated and written on a board, and then the sub-topics on adhesive notes are placed under the categories and then moved about and prioritized as necessary.

8. C: Increased nurse-to-patient ratio has been shown to consistently reduce hospital-associated adverse events. However, increasing the ratio is very costly. CMS currently requires only that hospitals have "adequate numbers" of licensed nurses but does not specify a ratio. California alone

225

has laws that require specific licensed nurse-to-patient ratios for different types of units while Massachusetts has a law regarding only ICU. Other states may require staffing committees or other approaches, such as public reporting of the ratio.

9. A: The type of leadership that is most likely to stifle creative problem-solving is bureaucratic. While this approach may be useful in handling financial matters or ensuring that safety procedures are following in dangerous situations, the bureaucratic leader is very rule-oriented and follows established protocols rather than looking toward creative solutions. Because others are expected to comply with all rules as well, staff members may be reluctant to offer innovative ideas, and opportunities for positive change may be lost.

10. D: Change theory (Lewin/Schein):

- Motivation to change (unfreezing): Dissatisfaction occurs and beliefs questioned, and survival anxiety may occur. Learning anxiety about having to learn different strategies causes resistance that can lead to denial, blame, and trying to maneuver or bargain without real change.
- Desire to change (unfrozen): Dissatisfaction is strong enough to override defensive actions. Desire to change is strong, but needed changes must be identified.
- Development of permanent change (refreezing): The new behavior becomes habitual, often requiring a change in perceptions of self and establishment of new relationships.

11. A: Emergency planning should begin with hazard vulnerability analysis, which assesses any potential hazards or threats that may impact the provision of care that must be maintained during an emergency situation. The primary vulnerabilities (flood, fire, terrorist attack, airline crash, chemical spill, nuclear reactor accident) should be identified and plans formulated. A hazard vulnerability analysis should be done on an annual basis and emergency preparedness plans updated according to the results of the analysis.

12. B: An operational database is generally utilized to track such things as inventory, purchases, patient information, and all financial transactions. Hierarchical databases are organized in a tree or parent-child formation with one piece of information connected to many (one-to-many), but in descending order only (not many-to-one). Relational databases are built on a multiple table structure with each individual item on a table having a unique identifier. Relational databases allow both one-to-many and many-to-one relationships. Real-time databases are used for rapidly changing data, such as stock market reports.

13. C: If the purpose of a project is to develop a new emergency preparedness plan, the document that is provided at the end of the project would be categorized as a deliverable. Deliverables are the end-products or services that are produced during different project phases. For example, the deliverable for the first project phase may be an annotated review of the current policy. The project plan should clearly outline the deliverables expected at each phase and the time frame.

14. B: If utilizing the Lean-Six Sigma approach (which combines Six Sigma with "lean" thinking) to performance improvement, the primary focus should be on strategic goals. The program aims to provide continuous learning and rapid change to reduce error and waste. Characteristics include:

- Long term goals and strategies for 1- to 3-year periods.
- Performance improvement as the underlying belief system.
- Cost reduction through quality increase.
- Incorporation of improvement methodology, such as DMAIC, PDCA, or other methods.

15. A: If the organization's overall staff turnover rate exceeds the benchmark (<6%) set by the organization, the next step should be to analyze the rate by job class. If, for example, the data is 9% staff turnover in nursing and 4% to 6% in other job classes, then strategies for retention need to be focused on nursing rather than on the other job classes. At this point, surveys and interviews should be carried out to obtain more data about nursing and focus groups formed.

16. D: If two members dominate team meetings, other members are likely to become bored or resentful, leading to an ineffective team. If this occurs, the leader must control the discussion and ensure that all members are heard and respected. Other characteristics of ineffective teams include autocratic leadership, unclear objectives, judgmental behavior, formal voting rather than consensus, and personal criticism rather than constructive. Members may try to avoid further conflict by suppressing opinions or feelings.

17. A: The measures presented in a balanced scorecard should be based on the organization's mission, vision, goals, and objectives as outlined in the strategic plan. The balanced scorecard may include financial data as well as data about customers, processes, and education, depending on the organization's needs. The balanced scorecard should reflect needs and priorities of the organization (clinical outcomes, growth initiatives, in-service, business operations, types of customer) as well as those of the community and customers.

18. C: The tool that may be used to best develop and manage a timeline for a quality improvement project is a GANTT chart. The GANTT chart is a bar chart that provides a visual representation of the timeline. Tasks are listed vertically on the left with horizontal bars (often color-coded) from the beginning point of a task to the ending point. Many tasks may overlap while some tasks may need to be completed before other tasks can begin.

19. B: If one unit in the hospital that has a far lower rate of hospital-associated infections than similar units is used as a performance indicator for comparison, this is an example of <u>internal benchmarking</u>. <u>Functional benchmarking</u> compares performance with similar organizations or those with similar challenges. <u>Generic benchmarking</u> compares business functions that are common to many different types of organizations. <u>Competitive benchmarking</u> compares measures from direct competitors, such as a hospital of similar size and services.

20. D: When using a run chart with more than 21 data points, variations include:

- <u>Trend</u>: 7 or more consecutive data points in ascending or descending order.
- <u>Run</u> (shift): ≥7 data consecutive data points all above or all below the median (run chart) or mean (control chart).
- <u>Cycle</u>: Up and down variation forming a sawtooth pattern with 14 successive data points, suggestive of systemic effect on data. If the trend is related to common cause variation, the variation may be demonstrated with 4-11 successive data points.
- <u>Astronomical value</u>: Data point unrelated to other points indicates sentinel event or special cause variation.

21. C: Third party payers, such as insurance companies, are most likely to assess the quality of patient care based on cost-effectiveness because their concern is to pay less for care. In some cases, this means that insurance companies are sometimes restrictive in what they are willing to pay for and may, for example, refuse to pay for costly treatments if less expensive treatments are available even if the less expensive treatments are also less effective.

22. B: CMS contracts with nongovernmental quality improvement organizations (QIOs), whose job is to monitor patient care by retrospective review of patient records. The records are reviewed to determine if they meet necessary criteria: medical necessity, appropriate level of care, and quality provision of care. Core functions of QIOs include improving health care, protecting Medicare funds, and protecting beneficiaries by addressing complaints and violations of EMTALA or other regulations.

23. A: A scattergram is a type of graphic display of the relationship between 2 variables with one variable plotted from the X axis and one from the Y axis. With enough data, patterns may begin to emerge. In a scattergram, if the data begin to form a straight-line pattern, this is evidence that there is a correlation between the two variables. The scattergram can be used to test for possible cause-effect relationships although this type of relationship is not required, and the scattergram alone is not proof of a correlation between data.

24. C: Based on HHS guidelines for pandemic planning, if 500,000 people in the local population fall ill, 50% of this group (250,000) are likely to seek outpatient medical care. This may result in a huge influx of patient to emergency rooms, doctor's offices, and clinics, most of which will not initially have adequate supplies of vaccines or antiviral medications. The death rate is dependent on the severity of the infection and the virulence of the virus.

25. B: Sixty-eight percent (68%) of data points normally fall with one standard deviation of the mean. The normal distribution of data follows the traditional bell curve and the 68-95-99 rule with 68% within the first standard deviation, 95% within the first and second, and 99% within the first, second, and third. Standard deviation allows the researcher to determine if data are typical of expected variation (falling within the 3 standard deviations) or are statistically significant (falling outside).

26. B: The type of error in measurement may occur if the participant reacts to the interviewer's lack of friendliness is situational contamination. That is, something in the situation or environment affects the outcome of measurement. This can include the mere presence of the interviewer (reactivity reaction) or such things as the temperature of the room, the lighting, and the ambient sound. Measurement should always be done with as few environmental distractions as possible.

27. D: The primary goal of the continuum of care is to provide healthcare to the point of optimal health. That is, healthcare should be provided as part of the continuum of care as long as it provides benefit. This encompasses not only personal care but laboratory testing and imaging, and medications. Healthcare provided that no longer provides any benefit, such as extensive treatments at the end of life, add to the financial burden of healthcare without return.

28. C: The semi-interquartile range (SIQR) method of determining variability eliminates the upper 25% and lower 25% of data and uses only the middle 50% of data. This prevents extreme outlier scores from adversely affecting the data computations. However, using only 50% of data may provide a skewed analysis. SIQR tends to provide a more accurate estimation of variability than range alone, but both provide less information than standard deviation, which includes all data.

29. A: If as part of a research project, an analysis of the null hypothesis results in a p-value of 0.001, this suggests that the null hypothesis is wrong because the p-value is equal to or less than 0.05. If the p-value were greater than 0.05, the null hypothesis cannot be rejected. If the p-value is close to 0.05, then the results are inconclusive. P-values, which fall between 0 and 1, help the reviewer to assess the strength of the evidence.

30. D: According to force field analysis (Lewin), the two forces that must be considered for change include:

- <u>Driving forces:</u> These are forces responsible for instigating and promoting change, such as leaders, incentives, and competition.
- <u>Restraining forces:</u> These are forces that resist change, such as poor attitudes, hostility, inadequate equipment, or insufficient funds.

Both forces must be considered when promoting change and a plan developed to diminish or eliminate restraining forces. A balance between forces represents the *status quo* or equilibrium.

31. B: If the process improvement team leader assigns a team facilitator, that individual's role is to manage conflicts and group dynamics. The team facilitator should be very familiar with the process improvement process as well as the target process or processes for the team and should ensure that the process improvement process is carried out effectively. The facilitator may also serve in the role of coach and/or mentor for other team members and serve as a consultant or advisor.

32. C: If the hospital has established a goal of reducing pressure sores by establishing and monitoring set time periods for turning patients, this represents a tertiary health promotion/preventative strategy:

- <u>Primary</u>: Specific preventive interventions, such as immunizations, use of safety glasses, fluoridation of water, and changing habits (smoking, drinking, diet) to prevent disease.
- <u>Secondary</u>: Screening to identify risks or disease (STDs, diabetes, hypertension) so preventive measures can be started to prevent progression of disease.
- <u>Tertiary</u>: Interventions to promote recovery and prevent disabilities, such as turning patients to prevent pressure sores and enrolling patients in rehabilitation programs.

33. A: The Agency for Healthcare Research and Quality (AHRQ) provides quality indicators (measures of quality in healthcare):

- <u>Prevention Quality Indicators:</u> Help to identify conditions in ambulatory care patients that can be addressed to prevent hospitalization or disease complications.
- <u>Patient Safety Indicators:</u> Help to identify potential adverse events and incidence of adverse events in patients after childbirth and invasive procedures.
- <u>Inpatient Quality Indicators:</u> Help to assess care and potential problems in inpatient care.
- <u>Pediatric Quality Indicators:</u> Help to identify and prevent complications and iatrogenic events in hospitalized pediatric patients.

34. B: According to the National Quality Forum (NQF), if a patient dies from a fall while hospitalized, this type of serious reportable event (SRE) would be reported as an environmental event. Other environmental events include death or serious injury disability associated with burns, use of restraints or bedrails, or electric shock as well as delivery of wrong or contaminated gas in oxygen or other gas line. SREs also include surgical events, product or device events, patient protection events, care management events, radiologic events, and potential criminal events.

35. D: According to the Institute of Health (IHI), the four criteria for Always Events are:

- <u>Important:</u> Based on patient identification of that which is most important to their care experience.
- <u>Evidence-based:</u> Research shows that the event (intervention) contributes positively to patient care and respect for patients.
- <u>Measurable:</u> Presence or absence of the event can be measured.
- <u>Affordable/Sustainable:</u> Ability to provide event without undue costs, new equipment, or capital outlay.

36. B: When conducting education or training programs for adults, it's important to remember that, according to the Theory of Andragogy (Knowles), adult learners tend to be:

- <u>Self-directed:</u> Provide overviews, summaries, problem-solving exercises.
- <u>Practical and goal-oriented:</u> Encourage input, give responsibilities, and allow opportunities.
- <u>Knowledgeable:</u> Show respect for life experience/education.
- <u>Relevancy oriented:</u> Identify objectives clearly.
- <u>Motivated:</u> Provide tangible reward for achievement.

37. A: Immunizations that the CDC currently recommends for all healthcare workers includes hepatitis B and influenza (annually). Other recommended immunizations include:

- MMR (measles, mumps, rubella): Two-dose series with second immunization at least 28 days after first for those born after 1957 and those born before 1957 without proof of immunity.
- Varicella (chicken pox): Two doses, four weeks apart.
- Tdap (tetanus, diphtheria, and pertussis): One time with tetanus (TD) booster every 10 years.
- Meningococcal: One dose.

38. C: The primary problem with assessing performance through direct observation is that performance may change under observation. Individuals tend to comply with rules and protocols more readily when observed and may work more slowly and methodically to ensure everything is done correctly, so workarounds and shortcuts that the individuals normally use may not be evident. Therefore, multiple assessment methods should be employed, such as anonymous surveys that includes questions about workarounds the individuals have used or have observed others using.

39. C: Preadmission services should base admission criteria on possible diagnosis. The care plan should begin at this point and may include contact not only with the physician who initiates the preadmission processes but with the patient who provides additional necessary information. Patients should be informed at this time if they are outside of the provider list and will have additional costs. Preadmission services may include contacting insurance carriers for preauthorization for treatments or procedures, based on the diagnosis.

40. D: A quality circle usually comprises 10 to 15 people supported by administration who serve on a committee that continually works toward quality improvement by evaluating processes, identifying and solving problems, and proposing ideas for improvement. The quality circle should include key individuals in the organization who are not only skilled and forward looking but who can influence other staff members to support quality improvements. The quality circle helps to guide and support process improvement implementation.

41. A: If a sample is obtained by enrolling all patients who come to an outpatient clinic until the target number of participants is reached, the type of sampling utilized is convenience (AKA accidental) sampling. This is the weakest form of sampling because it does not control for biases, and samples may not be adequately representative of the target population. However, this type of sampling is easy to do and inexpensive, and samples can usually be obtained quite quickly.

42. B: If, for clinical research regarding patient concerns, staff nurses in multiple departments will be provided questionnaires to administer to patients, the biggest concern regarding this method of data collection is likely consistency, a critical factor. For example, patients may be more alert and responsive in the morning than in the evening or may be less inclined to answer if in pain or tired. Nurses may use different approaches with patients, resulting in more or less cooperation. Training is, therefore, an important element.

43. D: Customers ultimately define organizational quality, which is dependent on their experience of care and perceptions. Regardless of accreditation or staff commitment to quality care, if patients have negative experiences, this can result in a public perception of inadequate care. This, in turn, may result in patients seeking care elsewhere. For this reason, it's especially important to include input from patients and key stakeholders in the community when developing quality improvement measures and to establish open communication.

44. C: When designing educational activities, the first step is to determine the purpose:

- Awareness: New regulations, Medicare laws, reimbursement concerns, changes in insurance coverage.
- Knowledge: New medications/ equipment, treatments, approaches to care, information about diseases.
- Safety: Use of safety equipment, fall prevention, immunization guidelines.
- Legal issues: Sexual harassment, bias, negligence, informed consent, end-of-life care, confidentiality and privacy (HIPAA).
- Clinical skills: Use of new equipment, insertion of PICC lines, physical assessment, ECG training.

45. B: FOCUS methodology for quality improvement:

- Find: Identifying a problem by looking at the organization and attempting to determine what errors in processes are occurring.
- Organize: Identifying those people who have an understanding of the problem or process and creating a team process improvement team.
- Clarify: Utilizing brainstorming techniques, such as the Ishikawa diagram, to better understand problems.
- Uncover: Analyzing the situation to determine the reason the problem has arisen or that a process is unsuccessful.
- Start: Determining where to begin in the change process.

46. A: When planning a staff meeting to discuss quality improvement initiatives, the CPHQ should first develop the agenda, ensuring that the agenda items fit into the allotted timeframe and allowing time for questions and discussions. The agenda should be sent out with the meeting announcements so that participants have some understanding of the purpose of the meeting and the topics of discussion. This allows the participants to come to the meeting better prepared.

47. C: The primary disadvantage of mailed surveys is that the return rate is low, often as low as 10 to 20%. Notifying potential participants in advance may help to increase the return rate, especially with digital surveys that can be easily completed and submitted. Email surveys are less expensive and should be designed so that they are easy to answer (such as by selecting the appropriate response rather than writing in information) and the data are easily quantifiable.

48. B: When facilitating quality improvement, the biggest barrier to implementation of changes is usually staff resistance to change. People develop a sense of security with familiarity, and new approaches, even though they may be demonstrably better, can result in anxiety and insecurity. Some people may feel that the changes suggests that they were less than competent before, and others may resent the time and effort needed to learn new skills or ways of doing things.

49. D: As part of performance improvement, the Ishikawa (fishbone) diagram may be used to help to identify root causes. The "head" is usually labeled with the problem (effect) and the bones with the causes, coded according to type:

- M (manufacturing): methods, materials, manpower, machines, measurement, mother nature (environment).
- P (administration and service): people, prices, promotion, places, policies, procedures, product.
- S (services): surroundings, suppliers, systems, skills.

50. A: When making a process map as part of needs assessment, the CPHQ must map the process as it actually takes place, not as it should or will with changes. This means, that the process should be mapped during direct observations and surveys, taking note of any work-arounds or shortcuts that are utilized. People often inaccurately report steps in a process. The process map should include times, such as the time needed to obtain supplies, and the complete cycle time from beginning to end.

51. C: If, when monitoring a quality improvement project, the CPHQ notes that all deliverables have been consistently behind schedule for the past 8 weeks, the best initial approach is to adjust the timeline. When creating the timeline, some extra time should be built in to allow for delays, and the initial timeline may have underestimated the time necessary. However, once the timeline is adjusted, CPHQ should try to identify weak links that are interfering with progress.

52. D: A complete history and physical examination should be completed on an inpatient with no recent history of care within 24 hours of admission. If the patient has had a history and physical completed in the 30 days prior to admission, only an update is required, but it should also be completed within 24 hours. The nursing assessment should be completed as well within 24 hours as it is the basis for the care plan. A functional assessment should be carried out along with the nursing assessment within the 24-hour timeframe.

53. B: The Plan-Do-Check-Act (PDCA) (Shewhart cycle) method of continuous quality improvement is best suited for specific problems rather than complex or organization-wide problems. PDCA is simple and easy to understand. Steps:

- Plan: Identify problem, set goals and establish process with brainstorming and data collection.
- Do: Generate solutions and pick one for a trial.
- Check: Analyze data and either continue or pick a different solution to implement.
- Act: Identify necessary changes, adopt, and continue to monitor.

54. D: If a "never event" occurs, the initial response should be to conduct a root-cause analysis to try to determine what problems in the system or processes may have led to the event. The focus should not be on assigning blame. Root cause analysis may include interviews, observations, and review of medical records. Often, an extensive questionnaire is completed by the professional doing the RCA, tracing essentially every step in the patient's hospitalization and care, including every treatment, every medication, and every contact.

55. A: If a hospital is interesting in applying for the Magnet Recognition Program® through the ANCC, the first step is to conduct a gap analysis to identify areas that need improvement. Magnet® status requires compliance with 14 "forces of magnetism" to demonstrate excellence in nursing care. Nursing CNOs must have an MS or doctorate and nurse managers at least a BSN. Additionally, the hospital should show progress toward a goal of 26% certification of the professional nursing staff. The hospital must show evidence of innovative health care, positive patient satisfaction, and good patient outcomes.

56. C: An innovation adopter who doesn't propose innovations but is willing to readily adopt them when proposed by others would be categorized as early majority. Types of innovation adopters:

- Innovators: First to seek and accept innovations and change. Often actively seek new information.
- Early adopters: Don't seek out innovations but recognize them and apply to practice. Often effective at communicating the value of innovations.
- Early majority: (As explained in answer explanation above.)
- Late majority: Reluctant to accept changes. Often must be pressured to overcome resistance.
- Laggards: Most resistant. Feel comfortable with the *status quo*.

57. B: DNV Global (DNV GL) is an accreditation organization for hospitals, critical access hospitals, and ancillary services (home health agencies, hospices, pharmacies, private duty, and DMEPOS). Certificates recognize expertise in managing of various conditions and include Managing Infection Risk, Primary Stroke Center, Comprehensive Stroke Center, Acute Stroke Ready, and Hip and Knee Replacement Program. DNV GL utilizes National Integrated Accreditation for Healthcare (NIAHO®) requirements and integrates CMS Conditions of Participation with ISO 9001 Quality Management program.

58. A: The primary purpose of rapid cycle testing is to reduce the time needed for implementation. Small scale tests are used to assess small sample sizes in a series of PDCA cycles that aim to identify both positive and negative results quickly so that modifications can be carried out. For example, a small number of staff members may test a process, or a process may be carried out for only a few days and then evaluated. Rapid cycle testing can drastically cut the time needed for implementation.

59. D: ISO 9000, published by the International Organization for Standardization (ISO), includes standards for quality management and promotes a process approach utilizing the PDCA cycle. Organizations wanting to utilize the standards purchase them from ISO. ISO 9001:2015 establishes necessary criteria for quality management with a focus on quality management principles: customer focus, leadership, engagement of people, process approach, evidence-based decision making, and relationship management.

60. B: The appropriate initial response if the hospital has received an onsite OSHA inspection because of a complaint filed by a worker about safety concerns is to take steps to remedy this safety concern. Complaints are kept anonymous to encourage people to report their concerns, so no efforts should be made to try to identify the worker. A later step may include calling a staff meeting to discuss safety concerns and assuring workers that any complaints or concerns will be addressed without retaliation.

61. C: The first step that must be carried out for an organization utilizing the Baldridge Excellence Framework to promote excellence is to create an organization profile. This provides an overview of the organization and should help to identify any gaps in information or performance. The organization profile includes the key descriptions of the organization:

- Organizational environment: Services, mission, vision, goals, workforce profile, assess, and regulatory requirements.
- Organizational relationships: Structure, patient and other customers and stakeholders, suppliers and partners.

62. A: Preparation for Joint Commission accreditation inspections should be carried out on a continuous basis so that the organization always remains in compliance and current with all new standards. Therefore, it's important that all staff members be educated about new standards and any changes in procedures or documentation resulting from the standards. Since 2006, inspections in the United States are unannounced, so managers across the organization must be in a state of constant readiness.

63. D: If an outbreak *Clostridium difficile* has occurred resulting in multiple cases of severe diarrhea in hospitalized patients and staff members on one unit, the initial infection control efforts should be aimed at hand washing procedures. The *C. diff* spores are very resistant and can survive for long periods on environmental surfaces. They are most often spread from one patient to another through contaminated hands. Older patients and those on long-term antibiotics are especially at risk.

64. C: If a patient satisfaction survey covers topics clearly related to issues of patient satisfaction, the type of validity the survey has is content validity. Discriminant validity is the degree of difference that occurs in the results if the measure is utilized in different settings. Criterion validity is the degree to which the scale correlates with another reliable scale. Convergent validity is the degree to which the scale shows a correlation between related item, such as wait time and satisfaction with service.

65. B: According to the Pyramid of Evidence (Haynes), AKA the 5 S's, a meta-analysis is categorized under syntheses. Pyramid:

- Studies (base): Qualitative studies, quantitative studies, case studies, and concept analyses.
- Syntheses: Systematic reviews, meta-analyses, literature reviews, integrative reviews.
- Synopses: Brief descriptions of research projects and studies.
- Summaries: More detailed descriptions of research projects and studies.
- Systems (point): EHRs integrated with practice guidelines.

Studies and syntheses carry the most weight when developing evidence-based guidelines and pathways.

66. D: To ensure that new hires are correctly licensed and credentialed, it is necessary to carry out a primary source verification. That means that sealed transcripts must be obtained for academic credits and certifying agencies contacted directly. It's also important to obtain copies of current license and credentials and to contact previous employers although privacy constraints limit the information employers can provide. A credential verification organization may be contracted to carry out verifications.

67. A: A process improvement team comprised only of members from one department or service area is categorized as a functional team. A functional team may or may not also be *ad hoc* (temporary) depending on the goals of the team, but most are permanent and led by a manager of the department or service area. Functional teams often meet on a regular schedule to review department/service issues and processes and to make suggestions for changes or improvements.

68. B: An appropriate narrative documentation is: "Patient states that he has not received assistance with bathing or dental care." While the patient may be unhappy, complaining, and wanting more care, this information alone does not describe what the real problem is, only the results of the problem. Documentation should always be as concrete as possible and should incorporate the patient's own statements into the report. Documentation should also include the steps taken to resolve the problem.

69. C: The four core criteria for credentialing and privileging include:

- Licensure: Must be current through the appropriate state board, such as state medical board.
- Education: Includes training and experience appropriate for the credential and may include technical training, professional education, residencies, internships, fellowships, doctoral and post-doctoral programs, and board and clinical certifications.
- Competence: Evaluations and recommendations by peers regarding clinical competence and judgment.
- Performance ability: Demonstrated ability to perform the duties to which the credentialing/privileging applies.

70. D: Test-retest reliability coefficient is a method used to measure instrument reliability. If information is unlikely to change, a retest of the same material should render the same results if the test is administered to the same individuals at different times. If the results vary, then the test lacks reliability and must be reassessed. If test-retest involves memory retrievable (such as a test of learned content); however, some degradation is expected because of limitations in short-term memory.

71. A: The most important element of a disaster/emergency preparedness plan is being readily available and having practice drills. Because disaster/emergency situations are generally rare, staff members may not recall how to activate the plan and carry out procedures unless they have had frequent opportunities to review the plan and practice. Disaster/emergency preparedness drills should be carried out at least annually and the plan updated, especially the chain of command and "phone tree" (including text or email) to reflect current staffing.

72. D: Medical orders for behavioral restraints for individuals ages 9 through 17 are time-limited to two hours, while for those under 9 are limited to one hour, and for those 18 and over, to four hours. Behavioral restraints should be avoided if at all possible and removed as soon as the patient reaches criteria for discontinuation. Patients younger than 17 must be reassessed for continued need for restraints at least every 4 hours, and those 18 and over, every 8 hours.

73. B: If data include patients' blood pressures, these data are categorized as continuous data because the values may vary widely. Continuous data may include decimal values within an established range. This type of data can be plotted on a scale or continuum. Other examples of continuous data include patient's weight, height, and temperature. Continuous data are usually plotted between maximum and minimum values (the range of values). Every point of plotted continuous data has meaning.

74. C: Principles of high-reliability organizations include:

- Constant concern regarding failure, constantly on alert.
- Focus on promoting organizational resilience, responding quickly to problems and errors.
- Attention to operations and allowing some autonomy to solve problems.
- Adequate communication with documentation standards adhered to.
- Promotion of culture or safety with reporting of problems rewarded.

75. A: When evaluating Internet sources as part of literature review and research, the two most important criteria are:

- Content: Consider the message, intention, juried/non-juried, type of content, and date.
- Credibility: Look for author's credentials, credible content, appropriate URL extension (.edu, .gov, .org, .net., .info).

The ten Cs for evaluating internet sources also include critical thinking, copyright, citation, continuity, censorship, connectivity, comparability, and context.

76. D: *PubMed* is the abstract database of the National Library of Medicine with millions of citations covering material from the 1950s to the present. *OVID* is a search platform that can be used to access a number of databases, including *Medline* and *CINAHL*, but requires subscription or payment. *EBSCO* is a search platform similar to *OVID* but requires institutional subscription. *CINAHL* is a nursing and allied health abstract database that includes materials from 1982 to the present.

77. B: Public perception of a hospital is important, and patients should not receive "surprise bills." Patients should be notified in advance when out-of-network providers are used and given estimates of cost before service is provided. Patients should also be provided information about alternatives if they are available. While state laws vary, patients may be able to file a complaint through the state's consumer protection agencies if they did not receive advance notice about out-of-network costs.

78. C: It the data set includes 68, 82, 86, 89, 90, 90, 91, 91, 92, 92 and 94, the median value is 90. When the data are placed in ascending order, the date point in the middle is the median. Median may be more accurate than mean because of outliers. For example, the mean of the 11 numbers above is 965/11 = 87.7. However, only 3 number fall below that average while 8 numbers fall above. The outlier of 68 gives an inaccurate picture of the data while the median (90) is a more accurate reflection.

79. D: If the CPHQ has determined that the hospital can better improve trauma care with the data provided by a trauma registry, the next step is to develop the case definition. The case definition usually includes the specific trauma diagnostic codes that will be included in the registry. Once the registry is established and the case definition completed, the CPHQ may develop protocols for case finding and submission of data, including the specific data elements that are to be included.

80. A: The primary purpose of the Healthcare Effective Data and Information Set (HEDIS) tool is to measure performance of over 80 measures in 5 domains of care: effectiveness of care, access/availability of care, experience of care, utilization and risk adjusted utilization, and relative resource. The data provided by HEDIS may be then utilized to reduce costs by identifying cost-effective interventions, set performance goals, and assess best practices. HEDIS data are collected from health plans and physicians and compiled in databases.

81. B: As with any changes in procedures or policies, the staff should be provided detailed guidelines and training of each element of SBAR as well as worksheets they can use to organize information. Elements include:

- Situation: Name, age, MD, diagnosis.
- Background: Brief medical history, co-morbidities, review of lab tests, current therapy, IV's, VS, pain, special needs, educational needs, discharge plans.
- Assessment: Review of systems, lines, tubes, and drains, completed tasks, needed tasks, future procedures.
- Recommendations: Review plan of care, medications, precautions (restraints, falls), treatments, wound care.

82. C: Pay-for-performance programs are usually based on four types of quality measures:

- Performance: Based on carrying out practices demonstrated to improve health outcomes.
- Outcomes: Based on achieving positive outcomes (but does not always consider social or other variables that the healthcare provider cannot control).
- Patient experience (satisfaction): Based on patient's perceptions of care received and their satisfaction.
- Structures/Technology: Based on facilities and equipment used for care, and may reward some types of upgrades, such as an upgrade to an electronic health record.

83. D: According to the general systems theory, changed behavior would be classified as an output. The general systems theory involves a cycle that includes 4 elements:

- Input: This is what goes into a system in terms of energy or materials, such as knowledge and facts.
- Throughput/Processes: These are the actions that take place in order to transform input, such as lived experience.
- Output: This is the result of the interrelationship between input and processes, such as changed behavior.
- Feedback: This is information that results and can be used for evaluation of the system, such as praise and support.

84. D: A team is best described as individuals working together to carry out a specific activity. Teams generally have defined objectives and work together in an interdependent manner. Team members may have to commit to training and considerable time in carrying out the tasks needed. Effective teams are characterized by good working relationships and respect among members and a willingness to assist each other and to make decisions through consensus. Leadership may be shared or may shift from time to time.

85. C: According to Westrum's phases of safety culture, an organization that indicates a concern for safety and takes action when an accident occurs to prevent a recurrence is in the reactive phase. Phases:

- Pathological: Little concern about safety issues even with awareness that problems exist.
- Reactive: As above.
- Calculative: Prepared to manage hazards/problems as they occur.

- Proactive: Steps in place to anticipate problems that may occur.
- Generative: Safety culture throughout, from senior management on down.

86. B: After selecting a number of possible vendors for a complex upgrade of equipment and services, the next step is to develop a request for proposal. With the request for proposal, there may be considerable differences among the different vendors related to the types of equipment and the costs or services. A request for quotation, on the other hand, is usually submitted for products or services that are essentially the same or very similar with cost one of the deciding factors.

87. A: Under the Joint Commission's policies, suicide within 72 hours of discharge is a reviewable sentinel event. Sentinel events include safety events that result in death, permanent harm/disability, or severe temporary harm/disability. Sentinel events must be reviewed by the hospital and may, as well, be reviewed by TJC. Steps include disclosing the event to patient, family, and hospital administration as well as conducting a root cause analysis and taking corrective actions.

88. D: Gonorrhea, along with many other diseases such as syphilis, TB, and malaria, are reportable diseases that require a written report. State laws may vary slightly in reporting requirements, which are based on CDC guidelines. Different types of reporting are required, depending on the disease. Some, including rubeola and pertussis, must be reported by telephone. Only totals rather than individual cases must be reported for some diseases, such as varicella, mumps, and influenza.

89. C: A patient safety event that reaches the patient in some manner but does not result in harm to the patient is categorized as a no-harm event although it is cause for concern and review. An adverse event, on the other hand, results in harm or injury to the patient. A close call is a patient safety event that occurs but does not reach or effect the patient. A hazardous condition is a dangerous situation that increases the risk that an adverse event may occur.

90. A: Functional care is a nursing care delivery system that is most economical but fragments care. With functional nursing, care is divided among different staff members. For example, one nurse may give treatments, another may give medications, another may assess the patient's general condition, and nursing assistants take vital signs and provide personal care. This system takes an assembly-line approach to patient care and is efficient, but a holistic view of the patient is overlooked.

91. C: An algorithm outlines systematic procedures based on a patient's treatment response, such as for asthma care. For example, if a patient experiences an asthma attack, the first step is to provide a short-acting bronchodilator. If the wheezing subsides, the algorithm indicates that no further treatment is needed, but if the wheezing does not subside, then the algorithm outlines further treatments. Algorithms are based on best practices and standards of care.

92. D: When assessing quality performance, efficacy refers to the degree to which an intervention accomplishes desired patient outcomes. Appropriateness refers to the degree to which an intervention is relevant to and meets the needs of the patient. Effectiveness refers to the degree to which an intervention is applied correctly in order to achieve expected patient outcomes. Efficiency refers to the degree to which an intervention attains expected outcomes without undue effort or cost.

93. B: When assessing the core measure related to use of high-risk medications in the elderly, most data will likely be obtained from EHRs. The EHRs should contain lists of patient's current medications and history of medications and treatments, as well as orders for new medications.

These data sources provide more accurate and quantifiable information than surveys or interviews, which rely on honesty and memory, both of which may be faulty.

94. A: The primary component of a life safety management program is a fire prevention plan. Fire prevention should be addressed during initial construction and outfitting of all facilities as well as during ongoing operations. Standards for fire prevention efforts are set by the National Fire Protection Association. All fire detection and fire-fighting equipment must be inspected and tested in accordance with the Life Safety Code. The plan must include a fire response plan and outline training and fire drills.

95. C: If hospital administration mandates a change in skill mix to decrease the number of registered nurses in order to save costs and cope with a nursing shortage, the first step should be to determine the tasks that can be done by non-RNs. These tasks may include transporting patients, taking routine vital signs, assisting patients with personal care and ADLs, looking for equipment, and delivering laboratory specimens. The next step is to determine how many of these tasks are currently being done by RNs and how much time this involves because these hours could be replaced by non-RN staff.

96. D: In a just culture, if a nurse who misread a medication order and administered an incorrect dosage to a patient should be consoled and supported as this is a human error. The just culture differentiates among:

- Human error: Inadvertent actions, mistakes, or lapses in proper procedure—Consider processes, procedures, training, and/or design to determine the cause of the error, console and support.
- At-risk behavior: Unjustified risk, choice—Provide incentives for correct behavior and disincentives for incorrect, provide coaching.
- Reckless behavior: Conscious disregard for proper procedures--Take remedial action and/or punitive action.

97. A: For safety reasons, fire alarms routinely disengage door locks, but this poses a potential risk of infant/child abduction as a kidnapper may trigger the alarm in order to gain entrance. If the fire alarm sounds, then personnel must monitor entrances and exits until the children are safely evacuated or the alarm stops and locks re-engage. Areas with infants and children should have only one public entry that is within view of the nurse station and is monitored, such as by video.

98. C: The primary advantage of "smart pumps" over standard infusion pumps is error prevention. The pharmacy sets up specific libraries of drugs for different areas of the hospital, such as ICU and NICU with lists of medications and appropriate dosages that the healthcare provider programming the pump can choose from. If doses are outside of the preset parameters, an alert is given which may or may not be overridden, depending on programming. Because alerts are logged, the hospital can track dosages that were initially set incorrectly.

99. B: If a power outage delayed surgeries when the backup power system failed, this would be classified as a special cause variation. Special cause variations are random and cannot be predicted and generally don't require major system modification. The cause is usually easy to identify. With common cause variations, on the other hand, the variations are inherent to the process. For example, medications scheduled for 8 AM may be administered in a 30- minute window (15 minutes before and after) because of normal variations in work load, and narrowing this window may be quite difficult.

100. D: When establishing hospital standard measures, an appropriate benchmark for admitting patients for observation who actually meet criteria for inpatient admission is 0%. Incorrectly admitting patients for observation is a costly error for the hospital because of a lower reimbursement rate, but it may also delay treatment. Additionally, because the observation is not a qualifying stay, the patient may not reach the 3-day hospitalization needed to qualify for extended care.

101. B: When preparing data for display, text against a bright color (such as yellow) may be distracting to the viewer. It is harder for the eyes to process text from an illuminated screen than from paper, and this can result in blurring if the font is too small (less than 12) or if print fonts (such as Times New Roman) are utilized instead of digital fonts designed for the web, such as Verdana and Lucida Sans/Grande. Text should be broken up into small paragraphs and underlining used to highlight text rather than bolding or italics.

102. A: Once an evidence-based change has been implemented, the next critical element is to measure outcomes to determine how the change has impacted care, especially those elements that are important for reimbursement and reporting: rates of complications and sentinel events, length of stay, rates of re-hospitalization, and costs of care. After measures are evaluated and data collected, the outcomes should be widely disseminated throughout the organization.

103. C: According to Hospital Compare, the most common overall rating for hospitals is 3 stars (39% of hospitals that provide enough data to be rated). Less than two percent of hospitals receive the highest 5-star rating. The ratings are based on scores for seven different types of measures: mortality, safety of care, readmission, patient experience, effectiveness of care, timeliness of care, and efficient use of medical imaging. The hospital scores are compared with national averages and information on the site indicates if the hospital is above, the same as, or below national averages.

104. A: If one of the hospitals strategic goals is to enhance the organization's clinical capabilities, then the improvement project that would have priority is expanding the emergency department to become a trauma center. Trauma centers include specialized staff, including surgeons and other physicians, who are trained to deal with severe injuries, such as gunshot wounds and traumatic brain injuries. Trauma centers are often part of the emergency department and allow trauma patients to be treated rather than stabilized and transferred.

105. D: Patient/Population. PICOT format:

P	Patient/ Population	List important characteristics: 35-year-old male with low back pain.
I	Intervention/ Indicator	Explain the desired intervention under consideration: Acupuncture.
C	Comparison/ Control	List other possible interventions or alternatives: Surgery.
O	Outcome	Provide the desired measurable outcomes: Decreased pain levels (from 6–7 to 1–2) and increased mobility.
T	Time	Timeframe (if appropriate)

106. B: If present-on-admission indicators for diagnoses have been frequently overlooked for patients because of inadequate data collection and evaluation, the most likely impact for the organization is misclassification as complications. This, in turn, may negatively affect both hospital quality ratings and reimbursement. The organization must determine where the weak links in the admission process lie and take steps to more accurately identify present-on-admission conditions.

107. C: If utilizing the CRAF method to record minutes of meetings of the process improvement team, CRAF stands for conclusions, recommendations, actions, and follow-up. Minutes that are concise and summarize the main issue are more likely to be read and reviewed than lengthy minutes that cover every detail. The minutes should indicate areas of ambiguity or non-consensus. The action section of the minutes may outline long-term plans as well as activities that should be carried out prior to the next meeting.

108. A: To comply with OSHA regulations, a healthcare worker exposed to HIV through a needlestick must be monitored after exposure for at least 12 months. The healthcare worker should be tested for HIV status at 1 month, 6 months, and 12 months and provided post-exposure prophylaxis as indicated, generally with 3 or more antiretroviral drugs for 4 weeks. The healthcare worker must have informed consent and confidentiality ensured in accordance with HIPAA regulations.

109. B: The purpose of a data-flow diagram is to show how data flow into a system from external sources and from one process to another. The data-flow diagram provides a graphic representation of a system and all its processes. The data-flow diagram is a simplified flow chart that utilizes only 4 types of symbols: Square (source of data or external entity), rounded rectangle (process), arrow (direction of flow), and three-sided open rectangle (data storage).

110. A: Interpretability is the degree to which the user of data is able to understand the rationale behind the date and the outcomes. Reliability refers to the consistency. That is, the data measure the same thing in multiple settings. Validity is the degree to which the data measure that which was intended. Stability is the degree to which the measure of the same thing/person produces the same results. So, an instrument administered to a patient one day should yield similar results if administered a week later.

111. C: Considering safety concerns, increasing rates of heroin addiction in the area may most impact the security management of a hospital. When rates of addiction increase, the crime rate tends to increase also as addicts not only steal goods and money to pay for their addiction but also seek out places with drugs available in order to steal narcotics, such as hospitals and pharmacies. Addicts may engage in drug seeking behavior and appear in emergency rooms with various types of complaints of pain.

112. D: Juran, who specialized in quality management, believed that quality was both income-oriented and cost-oriented because quality usually costs less in the long-term and enhances income. Juran's "quality trilogy" comprises:

- Quality planning: Identify customers and their needs and developing products/services to meet those needs.
- Quality improvement: Developing processes that allow optimal production of the product/service.
- Quality control: Ensure the process can produce the product/service.

113. A: If a patient gives permission for a staff person to accompany her throughout her visit and takes notes of the experience, this is an example of patient shadowing. The observer should not interrupt the process and should remain as unobtrusive as possible because any variable entered into a process may affect outcomes. The patient must give permission for the shadowing and be apprised of the purpose. Patient shadowing may be followed by a patient interview to determine the patient's response to the observations made.

114. C: Water-stained ceiling tiles pose an increased risk of infection as they can harbor fungal spores. Any water staining or water leaks pose increased risk, and removal must be done with appropriate safety precautions. If surface mold is evident, then an infection control risk assessment must be carried out. Moisture meters may be used to evaluate water content (which should be less than 20% to discourage growth of organisms), and infrared cameras may detect hidden moisture.

115. B: The RACE method of dealing with a fire is frequently used in training staff to respond:

- R: Rescue any patients or others in immediate danger.
- A: Activate alarms to get help and notify the fire department.
- C: Confine the fire by closing doors and windows.
- E: Extinguish the fire (using the PASS procedure) and prepare to evacuate patients is necessary.

The PASS procedure is used for extinguishers and includes (P) pull the pin, (A) aim the nozzle at the fire, (S) squeeze the handle, and (S) spray toward the base of the fire.

116. C: To determine whether an applicant requesting clinical privileges has settled malpractice claims, the organization must query the National Practitioner Data Bank (NPDB), which also includes the Healthcare Integrity and Protection Data Bank (HIPDB):

- NPDB: Established by the Health Care Quality Improvement Act (1986) to keep records of actions taken against licensed healthcare providers, including malpractice, privileging actions, and professional society actions.
- HIPDB: Established by direction of Health Insurance Portability and Accountability Act (1996) to keep records and provide information about civil judgment, criminal judgments and licensing actions directed at healthcare providers.

117. D: If the Joint Commission grants contingent accreditation, the organization is generally subject to a follow-up survey in 30 days, by which time the organization should have taken steps to correct areas in which they are out of compliance. The 5 JC categories of accreditation include:

- Accreditation.
- Accreditation with follow-up survey: Survey within 30 days to 6 months.
- Contingent: As above.
- Preliminary denial: Organization may appeal and provide further data.
- Denial: No further appeal process is available.

118. C: Process improvement cycle:

- Initiation: Create mission and vision statements, define project, and form teams.
- Planning: Develop schedules and standards, estimate costs, identify activities, and develop training/implementation plans.
- Execution: Implement plan, start training, monitor progress, and evaluate and modify plan.
- Closure: Produce and disseminate final report and carry out ongoing evaluation.

119. A: In a PERT (Program Evaluation and Review Technique) chart, parallel activities occur at the same time. The PERT chart is a diagram that shows the sequence and duration of activities, with activities lettered sequentially starting with a, b, c... and the days needed for each activity are included by each letter. Lines and arrows connect the activities to show the direction of flow and which activities must be completed before others and which are done in parallel.

120. B: If implementing more streamlined procedures results in a lighter workload but elimination of some staff positions, the likely response to remaining staff will be anxiety. Whenever staff members see others losing their jobs, they fear that they will be next, regardless of reassurances from administration, especially if the job losses are in their department. It's important to provide advance notice and rationale for loss of positions to help allay fears and if possible, to reassign staff to other areas.

121. D: The first step in change management is to identify the losses that will occur. All change results in some type of loss as new policies and procedures are implemented, even if the changes are positive, so identifying these and then acknowledging them, providing information, and asking for feedback may help to alleviate fears that staff members may have about how the changes will affect them personally and professionally. The ending should be clearly marked in some way as well as the transition to the new beginning.

122. A: The four basic elements of malpractice include:

- <u>Duty to use due care:</u> Failure to meet standards set by law, contract, or standard practice.
- <u>Breach of duty:</u> An act of omission or commission.
- <u>Damages:</u> Harm that results, may be physical, emotional, or financial.
- <u>Causation:</u> Evidence that the breach of duty resulted in the damages.

In order to receive judgment for a plaintiff (the complainant), all four of these elements of malpractice must be proven.

123. C: Before construction begins on a renovation project, life safety and infection control assessments should be completed to evaluate the risk. The construction may negatively impact life safety codes if, for example, it increases the risk that a fire may occur. Additionally, if the construction generates dust, this can pose a considerable risk of infection to vulnerable patients. Also, if there is water damage, spores may be released, so the flow of air between the construction site and the rest of the facility must be carefully assessed.

124. B: Under tort law, a nurse who tells an uncooperative patient that he is being ridiculous and threatens to carry out a treatment on the patient against the patient's will may be charged with assault. Any threat to touch or harm a patient in some way without the patient's permission may be considered assault. Battery, on the other hand, is actually carrying out the act, such as (in this case) carrying out the treatment.

125. C: In the case of malpractice, peer review information (such as documents of discussion and decisions) is protected, which means the review documents are not admissible in court and, therefore, not discoverable, so as to encourage honest reviews. However, the members of the peer review committee can still be called to give testimony. Privileged information is that which cannot be divulged because of a special relationship, such as that between priest and confessor, married person and spouse, and lawyer and client.

126. D: In human factor engineering, forcing function refers to requiring a specific step before another step can be performed. For example, if dosage alerts on the EHR have been routinely ignored, the alerts may be programmed so that the person must click on a response before proceedings. Forcing function is done to prevent errors and improve safety measures. Another way to force function may be to remove certain drugs or equipment from nursing units and require special steps to obtain them, decreasing the risk that they may be used incorrectly.

127. A: According to Havelock's (1973) Six Phases of Planned Change, the first phase involves:

1. <u>Build relationship with the system</u>: Understand the system as it is and the dynamics and organizational culture.
2. <u>Diagnose problems</u>: Determine if change is indicated.
3. <u>Obtain necessary resources</u>: Recognize the need for change and begins to determine the resources needed.
4. <u>Select a solution</u>: Explore different options and choose one or more.
5. <u>Garner acceptance</u>: Monitor compliance and resistance.
6. Stabilize the change and facilitate self-renewal: Conduct ongoing monitoring.

128. B: If a nurse promises to check on a patient every hour and follows through on the promise, the nurse is exhibiting adherence to the ethical principle of <u>fidelity</u>, keeping one's word. <u>Veracity</u> is obligation to tell the truth. <u>Advocacy</u> refers to the obligation to stand up for the rights of others, such as patients, and top ensure they get the best care. <u>Beneficence</u> is the obligation to do good, especially in the provision of care.

129. D: The purpose of selecting a trigger for each measure of performance is to indicate when further analysis, such as root cause analysis or case review, needs to be carried out. Internal triggers may include sentinel events, performance rate, rate change, control limits, range of variation (by standard deviation methods), and differences between groups. External triggers may include staff and/or patient feedback, practice guidelines, benchmarks, research data, and strategic planning initiatives.

130. C: For staffing purposes, a staff nurse who works 20 hours a week throughout the year would be considered 0.5 FTE. FTE (full-time equivalent) is based on working 40 hours a week for 52 weeks a year (including paid sick time and vacation time). Those who work three 12-hour shifts (total 36 hours) are classified as 0.9 FTE even though they may be paid the full-time rate because the missing 4 hours must be covered by other personnel.

131. A: The first stage of strategic planning involves external and internal environment assessment:

- <u>External</u>: A broad analysis should include review of the political climate, economic standing, demographic factors, and technology. Additionally, the competition (such as other hospitals in the area) should be assessed and the likely impact of strategic planning initiatives on this competition.
- <u>Internal</u>: This analysis should cover all aspects of an organization, including resources in terms of buildings, technology, and resources (human and financial).

132. B: If a team leader states, "I am worried about nurse X's anger and hostility and wonder how I can help to reduce tension," the communication pattern the team member is using is congruence because the team leader's inner feelings ("worried") match the message ("help to reduce tension"). A pattern of placation results in trying to appease others while irrelevance results in changing the subject; and blame, pointing the finger at others.

133. D: An <u>unconscious reactive response</u>, such as blaming others, is based on feelings rather than rational thought or recognition of those feelings. Other unconscious reactive responses include making unreasonable demands on others, usually in response to anxiety or distress, or passing unfair judgments on others. With <u>conscious reactive responses</u>, the person recognizes and acknowledges personal feelings and thoughts, accepts accountability, and shows respect and compassion for others.

134. C: The most essential step in supply management is effective purchasing. This may involve negotiating for the best price and comparing different products and services to find the most cost-effective suppliers. In some cases, purchasing may involving participating in purchasing agreements with other organizations in order to obtain discounts only available for large orders. Effective purchasing also involves issuing request for information (RFI) to gain information from various vendors, often with request for quote (RFQ) or request for proposal (RFP).

135. B: The primary purpose of workflow analysis of processes is to identify bottlenecks or anything that impedes or interferes with the process. Bottlenecks may be individuals who are resistive to changes or undertrained or inadequate equipment. Bottlenecks may also be inherent to the process itself, such as redundant or confusing steps. Workflow analysis begins by outlining every step in the process and then carrying out observations and surveys to evaluate the process.

136. A: If a security breach involving a patient's EHR occurred when a nurse logged onto the EHR and then left the computer without logging out and a visitor read information on the computer screen, the best solution is to add an automatic log-off (timeout) feature. This feature locks the system after a prescribed period of time with no keyboard or mouse/trackpad activity. Unlocking the system requires logging in with an appropriate password.

137. D: A big bang implementation involves a complete new system going live at the same time across and organization, such as a switch from paper documentation to an EHR. Phased/Rollout implementation may involve phasing by module, unit, or geography rather than all at once. Pilot implementation tries out a new system in a smaller program, such as on one unit, before going system-wide. Parallel implementation involves use of both a new program and the old concurrently initially so users can learn the new system while still utilizing the old.

138. B: If information from patient EHRs has been shared with unauthorized individuals, the best approach to identifying how the breach occurred is to carry out audit trails. Audit trails are records of activity related to systems and software applications and traces user access and utilization. Audit trails can help to identify unauthorized users (such as a nurse accessing the record of a patient not under the nurse's care), equipment misuse, and attempted or successful penetration of the system.

139. C: When gathering data and assessing risks as part of the risk management team, the best approach is to use multiple measures, such as quantitative measures (questionnaires, record review), qualitative measures (narrative open-ended interviews), and observations. Individuals from multiple disciplines across the organizations and at different levels should be interviewed as perceptions may vary widely. The data should be utilized to produce action plans to resolve any problems areas identified through the assessment process.

140. C: Both expected changes and unexpected changes should be included in patients' discharge care plans:

Expected changes: Likely to occur and depend on the underlying condition and may include, for instance, plans to deal with increasing shortness of breath or increasing pain. The patient should be prepared in advance, knowing what to expect and what to do.

<u>Unexpected changes:</u> Unlikely, but may occur, such as wound infections, adverse effects of medications, and other complications. Patients should be aware of potential problems, taught to recognize them, and know how to deal with them, such as when to notify the physician.

How to Overcome Test Anxiety

Just the thought of taking a test is enough to make most people a little nervous. A test is an important event that can have a long-term impact on your future, so it's important to take it seriously and it's natural to feel anxious about performing well. But just because anxiety is normal, that doesn't mean that it's helpful in test taking, or that you should simply accept it as part of your life. Anxiety can have a variety of effects. These effects can be mild, like making you feel slightly nervous, or severe, like blocking your ability to focus or remember even a simple detail.

If you experience test anxiety—whether severe or mild—it's important to know how to beat it. To discover this, first you need to understand what causes test anxiety.

Causes of Test Anxiety

While we often think of anxiety as an uncontrollable emotional state, it can actually be caused by simple, practical things. One of the most common causes of test anxiety is that a person does not feel adequately prepared for their test. This feeling can be the result of many different issues such as poor study habits or lack of organization, but the most common culprit is time management. Starting to study too late, failing to organize your study time to cover all of the material, or being distracted while you study will mean that you're not well prepared for the test. This may lead to cramming the night before, which will cause you to be physically and mentally exhausted for the test. Poor time management also contributes to feelings of stress, fear, and hopelessness as you realize you are not well prepared but don't know what to do about it.

Other times, test anxiety is not related to your preparation for the test but comes from unresolved fear. This may be a past failure on a test, or poor performance on tests in general. It may come from comparing yourself to others who seem to be performing better or from the stress of living up to expectations. Anxiety may be driven by fears of the future—how failure on this test would affect your educational and career goals. These fears are often completely irrational, but they can still negatively impact your test performance.

Review Video: 3 Reasons You Have Test Anxiety
Visit mometrix.com/academy and enter code: 428468

247

Elements of Test Anxiety

As mentioned earlier, test anxiety is considered to be an emotional state, but it has physical and mental components as well. Sometimes you may not even realize that you are suffering from test anxiety until you notice the physical symptoms. These can include trembling hands, rapid heartbeat, sweating, nausea, and tense muscles. Extreme anxiety may lead to fainting or vomiting. Obviously, any of these symptoms can have a negative impact on testing. It is important to recognize them as soon as they begin to occur so that you can address the problem before it damages your performance.

> **Review Video: 3 Ways to Tell You Have Test Anxiety**
> Visit mometrix.com/academy and enter code: 927847

The mental components of test anxiety include trouble focusing and inability to remember learned information. During a test, your mind is on high alert, which can help you recall information and stay focused for an extended period of time. However, anxiety interferes with your mind's natural processes, causing you to blank out, even on the questions you know well. The strain of testing during anxiety makes it difficult to stay focused, especially on a test that may take several hours. Extreme anxiety can take a huge mental toll, making it difficult not only to recall test information but even to understand the test questions or pull your thoughts together.

> **Review Video: How Test Anxiety Affects Memory**
> Visit mometrix.com/academy and enter code: 609003

Effects of Test Anxiety

Test anxiety is like a disease—if left untreated, it will get progressively worse. Anxiety leads to poor performance, and this reinforces the feelings of fear and failure, which in turn lead to poor performances on subsequent tests. It can grow from a mild nervousness to a crippling condition. If allowed to progress, test anxiety can have a big impact on your schooling, and consequently on your future.

Test anxiety can spread to other parts of your life. Anxiety on tests can become anxiety in any stressful situation, and blanking on a test can turn into panicking in a job situation. But fortunately, you don't have to let anxiety rule your testing and determine your grades. There are a number of relatively simple steps you can take to move past anxiety and function normally on a test and in the rest of life.

> **Review Video: How Test Anxiety Impacts Your Grades**
> Visit mometrix.com/academy and enter code: 939819

Physical Steps for Beating Test Anxiety

While test anxiety is a serious problem, the good news is that it can be overcome. It doesn't have to control your ability to think and remember information. While it may take time, you can begin taking steps today to beat anxiety.

Just as your first hint that you may be struggling with anxiety comes from the physical symptoms, the first step to treating it is also physical. Rest is crucial for having a clear, strong mind. If you are tired, it is much easier to give in to anxiety. But if you establish good sleep habits, your body and mind will be ready to perform optimally, without the strain of exhaustion. Additionally, sleeping well helps you to retain information better, so you're more likely to recall the answers when you see the test questions.

Getting good sleep means more than going to bed on time. It's important to allow your brain time to relax. Take study breaks from time to time so it doesn't get overworked, and don't study right before bed. Take time to rest your mind before trying to rest your body, or you may find it difficult to fall asleep.

Review Video: The Importance of Sleep for Your Brain
Visit mometrix.com/academy and enter code: 319338

Along with sleep, other aspects of physical health are important in preparing for a test. Good nutrition is vital for good brain function. Sugary foods and drinks may give a burst of energy but this burst is followed by a crash, both physically and emotionally. Instead, fuel your body with protein and vitamin-rich foods.

Also, drink plenty of water. Dehydration can lead to headaches and exhaustion, especially if your brain is already under stress from the rigors of the test. Particularly if your test is a long one, drink water during the breaks. And if possible, take an energy-boosting snack to eat between sections.

Review Video: How Diet Can Affect your Mood
Visit mometrix.com/academy and enter code: 624317

Along with sleep and diet, a third important part of physical health is exercise. Maintaining a steady workout schedule is helpful, but even taking 5-minute study breaks to walk can help get your blood pumping faster and clear your head. Exercise also releases endorphins, which contribute to a positive feeling and can help combat test anxiety.

When you nurture your physical health, you are also contributing to your mental health. If your body is healthy, your mind is much more likely to be healthy as well. So take time to rest, nourish your body with healthy food and water, and get moving as much as possible. Taking these physical steps will make you stronger and more able to take the mental steps necessary to overcome test anxiety.

Review Video: How to Stay Healthy and Prevent Test Anxiety
Visit mometrix.com/academy and enter code: 877894

Mental Steps for Beating Test Anxiety

Working on the mental side of test anxiety can be more challenging, but as with the physical side, there are clear steps you can take to overcome it. As mentioned earlier, test anxiety often stems from lack of preparation, so the obvious solution is to prepare for the test. Effective studying may be the most important weapon you have for beating test anxiety, but you can and should employ several other mental tools to combat fear.

First, boost your confidence by reminding yourself of past success—tests or projects that you aced. If you're putting as much effort into preparing for this test as you did for those, there's no reason you should expect to fail here. Work hard to prepare; then trust your preparation.

Second, surround yourself with encouraging people. It can be helpful to find a study group, but be sure that the people you're around will encourage a positive attitude. If you spend time with others who are anxious or cynical, this will only contribute to your own anxiety. Look for others who are motivated to study hard from a desire to succeed, not from a fear of failure.

Third, reward yourself. A test is physically and mentally tiring, even without anxiety, and it can be helpful to have something to look forward to. Plan an activity following the test, regardless of the outcome, such as going to a movie or getting ice cream.

When you are taking the test, if you find yourself beginning to feel anxious, remind yourself that you know the material. Visualize successfully completing the test. Then take a few deep, relaxing breaths and return to it. Work through the questions carefully but with confidence, knowing that you are capable of succeeding.

Developing a healthy mental approach to test taking will also aid in other areas of life. Test anxiety affects more than just the actual test—it can be damaging to your mental health and even contribute to depression. It's important to beat test anxiety before it becomes a problem for more than testing.

Review Video: Test Anxiety and Depression
Visit mometrix.com/academy and enter code: 904704

Study Strategy

Being prepared for the test is necessary to combat anxiety, but what does being prepared look like? You may study for hours on end and still not feel prepared. What you need is a strategy for test prep. The next few pages outline our recommended steps to help you plan out and conquer the challenge of preparation.

STEP 1: SCOPE OUT THE TEST

Learn everything you can about the format (multiple choice, essay, etc.) and what will be on the test. Gather any study materials, course outlines, or sample exams that may be available. Not only will this help you to prepare, but knowing what to expect can help to alleviate test anxiety.

STEP 2: MAP OUT THE MATERIAL

Look through the textbook or study guide and make note of how many chapters or sections it has. Then divide these over the time you have. For example, if a book has 15 chapters and you have five days to study, you need to cover three chapters each day. Even better, if you have the time, leave an extra day at the end for overall review after you have gone through the material in depth.

If time is limited, you may need to prioritize the material. Look through it and make note of which sections you think you already have a good grasp on, and which need review. While you are studying, skim quickly through the familiar sections and take more time on the challenging parts. Write out your plan so you don't get lost as you go. Having a written plan also helps you feel more in control of the study, so anxiety is less likely to arise from feeling overwhelmed at the amount to cover.

STEP 3: GATHER YOUR TOOLS

Decide what study method works best for you. Do you prefer to highlight in the book as you study and then go back over the highlighted portions? Or do you type out notes of the important information? Or is it helpful to make flashcards that you can carry with you? Assemble the pens, index cards, highlighters, post-it notes, and any other materials you may need so you won't be distracted by getting up to find things while you study.

If you're having a hard time retaining the information or organizing your notes, experiment with different methods. For example, try color-coding by subject with colored pens, highlighters, or post-it notes. If you learn better by hearing, try recording yourself reading your notes so you can listen while in the car, working out, or simply sitting at your desk. Ask a friend to quiz you from your flashcards, or try teaching someone the material to solidify it in your mind.

STEP 4: CREATE YOUR ENVIRONMENT

It's important to avoid distractions while you study. This includes both the obvious distractions like visitors and the subtle distractions like an uncomfortable chair (or a too-comfortable couch that makes you want to fall asleep). Set up the best study environment possible: good lighting and a comfortable work area. If background music helps you focus, you may want to turn it on, but otherwise keep the room quiet. If you are using a computer to take notes, be sure you don't have any other windows open, especially applications like social media, games, or anything else that could distract you. Silence your phone and turn off notifications. Be sure to keep water close by so you stay hydrated while you study (but avoid unhealthy drinks and snacks).

Also, take into account the best time of day to study. Are you freshest first thing in the morning? Try to set aside some time then to work through the material. Is your mind clearer in the afternoon or evening? Schedule your study session then. Another method is to study at the same time of day that you will take the test, so that your brain gets used to working on the material at that time and will be ready to focus at test time.

STEP 5: STUDY!

Once you have done all the study preparation, it's time to settle into the actual studying. Sit down, take a few moments to settle your mind so you can focus, and begin to follow your study plan. Don't give in to distractions or let yourself procrastinate. This is your time to prepare so you'll be ready to fearlessly approach the test. Make the most of the time and stay focused.

Of course, you don't want to burn out. If you study too long you may find that you're not retaining the information very well. Take regular study breaks. For example, taking five minutes out of every hour to walk briskly, breathing deeply and swinging your arms, can help your mind stay fresh.

As you get to the end of each chapter or section, it's a good idea to do a quick review. Remind yourself of what you learned and work on any difficult parts. When you feel that you've mastered the material, move on to the next part. At the end of your study session, briefly skim through your notes again.

But while review is helpful, cramming last minute is NOT. If at all possible, work ahead so that you won't need to fit all your study into the last day. Cramming overloads your brain with more information than it can process and retain, and your tired mind may struggle to recall even previously learned information when it is overwhelmed with last-minute study. Also, the urgent nature of cramming and the stress placed on your brain contribute to anxiety. You'll be more likely to go to the test feeling unprepared and having trouble thinking clearly.

So don't cram, and don't stay up late before the test, even just to review your notes at a leisurely pace. Your brain needs rest more than it needs to go over the information again. In fact, plan to finish your studies by noon or early afternoon the day before the test. Give your brain the rest of the day to relax or focus on other things, and get a good night's sleep. Then you will be fresh for the test and better able to recall what you've studied.

STEP 6: TAKE A PRACTICE TEST

Many courses offer sample tests, either online or in the study materials. This is an excellent resource to check whether you have mastered the material, as well as to prepare for the test format and environment.

Check the test format ahead of time: the number of questions, the type (multiple choice, free response, etc.), and the time limit. Then create a plan for working through them. For example, if you have 30 minutes to take a 60-question test, your limit is 30 seconds per question. Spend less time on the questions you know well so that you can take more time on the difficult ones.

If you have time to take several practice tests, take the first one open book, with no time limit. Work through the questions at your own pace and make sure you fully understand them. Gradually work up to taking a test under test conditions: sit at a desk with all study materials put away and set a timer. Pace yourself to make sure you finish the test with time to spare and go back to check your answers if you have time.

After each test, check your answers. On the questions you missed, be sure you understand why you missed them. Did you misread the question (tests can use tricky wording)? Did you forget the information? Or was it something you hadn't learned? Go back and study any shaky areas that the practice tests reveal.

Taking these tests not only helps with your grade, but also aids in combating test anxiety. If you're already used to the test conditions, you're less likely to worry about it, and working through tests until you're scoring well gives you a confidence boost. Go through the practice tests until you feel comfortable, and then you can go into the test knowing that you're ready for it.

Test Tips

On test day, you should be confident, knowing that you've prepared well and are ready to answer the questions. But aside from preparation, there are several test day strategies you can employ to maximize your performance.

First, as stated before, get a good night's sleep the night before the test (and for several nights before that, if possible). Go into the test with a fresh, alert mind rather than staying up late to study.

Try not to change too much about your normal routine on the day of the test. It's important to eat a nutritious breakfast, but if you normally don't eat breakfast at all, consider eating just a protein bar. If you're a coffee drinker, go ahead and have your normal coffee. Just make sure you time it so that the caffeine doesn't wear off right in the middle of your test. Avoid sugary beverages, and drink enough water to stay hydrated but not so much that you need a restroom break 10 minutes into the test. If your test isn't first thing in the morning, consider going for a walk or doing a light workout before the test to get your blood flowing.

Allow yourself enough time to get ready, and leave for the test with plenty of time to spare so you won't have the anxiety of scrambling to arrive in time. Another reason to be early is to select a good seat. It's helpful to sit away from doors and windows, which can be distracting. Find a good seat, get out your supplies, and settle your mind before the test begins.

When the test begins, start by going over the instructions carefully, even if you already know what to expect. Make sure you avoid any careless mistakes by following the directions.

Then begin working through the questions, pacing yourself as you've practiced. If you're not sure on an answer, don't spend too much time on it, and don't let it shake your confidence. Either skip it and come back later, or eliminate as many wrong answers as possible and guess among the remaining ones. Don't dwell on these questions as you continue—put them out of your mind and focus on what lies ahead.

Be sure to read all of the answer choices, even if you're sure the first one is the right answer. Sometimes you'll find a better one if you keep reading. But don't second-guess yourself if you do immediately know the answer. Your gut instinct is usually right. Don't let test anxiety rob you of the information you know.

If you have time at the end of the test (and if the test format allows), go back and review your answers. Be cautious about changing any, since your first instinct tends to be correct, but make sure you didn't misread any of the questions or accidentally mark the wrong answer choice. Look over any you skipped and make an educated guess.

At the end, leave the test feeling confident. You've done your best, so don't waste time worrying about your performance or wishing you could change anything. Instead, celebrate the successful completion of this test. And finally, use this test to learn how to deal with anxiety even better next time.

Important Qualification

Not all anxiety is created equal. If your test anxiety is causing major issues in your life beyond the classroom or testing center, or if you are experiencing troubling physical symptoms related to your anxiety, it may be a sign of a serious physiological or psychological condition. If this sounds like your situation, we strongly encourage you to seek professional help.

Thank You

We at Mometrix would like to extend our heartfelt thanks to you, our friend and patron, for allowing us to play a part in your journey. It is a privilege to serve people from all walks of life who are unified in their commitment to building the best future they can for themselves.

The preparation you devote to these important testing milestones may be the most valuable educational opportunity you have for making a real difference in your life. We encourage you to put your heart into it—that feeling of succeeding, overcoming, and yes, conquering will be well worth the hours you've invested.

We want to hear your story, your struggles and your successes, and if you see any opportunities for us to improve our materials so we can help others even more effectively in the future, please share that with us as well. **The team at Mometrix would be absolutely thrilled to hear from you!** So please, send us an email (support@mometrix.com) and let's stay in touch.

> **If you'd like some additional help, check out these other resources we offer for your exam:**
> **http://MometrixFlashcards.com/CPHQ**

Additional Bonus Material

Due to our efforts to try to keep this book to a manageable length, we've created a link that will give you access to all of your additional bonus material.

Please visit http://www.mometrix.com/bonus948/cphq to access the information.